The Medical Assistant

CLINICAL PRACTICE

The Medical Assistant

CLINICAL PRACTICE

10 9 8

LIBRARY OF CONGRESS CATALOG CARD NUMBER: 76-5301
ISBN: 0-8273-0251-3

Printed in the United States of America
Published simultaneously in Canada
by Nelson Canada,
A Division of International Thomson Limited

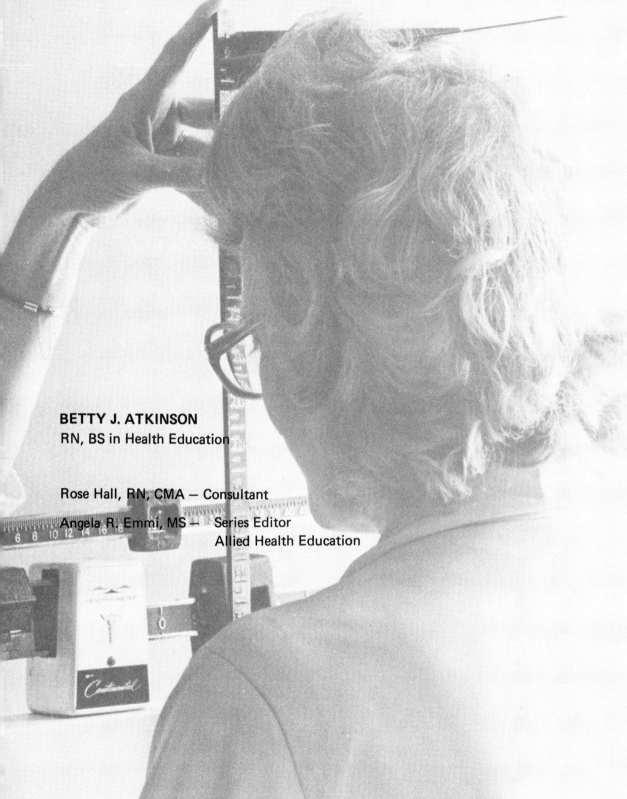

BETTY J. ATKINSON
RN, BS in Health Education

Rose Hall, RN, CMA — Consultant

Angela R. Emmi, MS — Series Editor
Allied Health Education

DELMAR PUBLISHERS INC.
2 COMPUTER DRIVE, WEST
BOX 15-015
ALBANY, NEW YORK 12212

Preface

The Medical Assistant-Clinical Practice can be used in the two-year medical assisting programs, private medical assistant schools, and in-service medical offices. It may complement texts that are currently available and/or be incorporated in a program of individualized instruction. It is designed to be used with guidance and resources provided by the instructor.

By carefully reading the objectives at the beginning of each unit, studying the text and following the suggested activities, the student should be able to perform well in the clinical area. Results of the unit reviews and sectional self-evaluation tests provide evidence of progress and achievement of mastery learning.

The Medical Assistant-Clinical Practice introduces the student medical assistant to the clinical setting and to the medical procedures which are necessary for her to perform independently and/or with the physician. The first portion of the text deals with basic skills involved with the assistant's first encounters with the patient. Gradually, the student learns about principles underlying aseptic technique and how to set up a sterile field in preparation for specific treatments and minor surgery. Proceeding to step-by-step descriptions of office procedures, the student advances to those treatments which require more responsibility. The administration of medications, venipuncture technique and the manner in which an electrocardiogram is taken are additional features which supplement instruction given by the physician, or another health professional.

Most of the units, especially those dealing with aseptic techniques, the administration of drugs, and venipunctures require basic instruction in the biological sciences and practical instruction by qualified personnel. *The medical assistant must never assume responsibility for anything she has not been taught to do, and authorized to perform by the physician.* A genuine concern for the safety of the patient, and freedom from possible legal action for the physician and the medical assistant must be present at all times.

Other features of *The Medical Assistant-Clinical Practice* include an appendix which presents an introduction to the specialty areas, charts with the normal values of various lab tests, facts about X rays, and a chart with the temperature conversion formula and comparable Fahrenheit-Centigrade readings.

The author, Betty Jean Atkinson, has a BS in Health Education and attended graduate school at Georgia Southwestern University. She designed a curriculum for medical office assistants and taught the program for several years. In addition to experience in the field of medical assisting, Ms. Atkinson has taught students of practical nursing and registered nursing. She also organized and operated a course of instruction for nurse technicians in a vocational rehabilitation center. Ms. Atkinson served as a research assistant in anatomy and physiology, and as a career consultant for the State Scholarship Commission in Atlanta, Georgia. She has worked closely with Manpower Development Training programs in Georgia.

Other Books in Delmar's health education series are:

Body Structure and Functions	Diversified Health Occupations
Microbiology for Health Careers	Health Assistant
Coping with Illness	Fundamental Mathematics for Health Careers
Understanding Human Behavior	Geriatrics
Dental Assistant	Mental Health Concepts

Contents

SECTION 6 OTHER DIAGNOSTIC PROCEDURES

SECTION 7 EMERGENCIES

APPENDIX

Cardiology and Internal Medicine
Dermatology and Allergy
Ear, Nose, and Throat
Endocrinology
Gerontology
Neurology
Obstetrics and Gynecology
Ophthalmology
Orthopedics
Pediatrics
Psychiatry
Surgery
Urology

Section 1 The Medical Assistant and the Patient

Unit 1 Role of the Medical Assistant

OBJECTIVES

After studying this unit, the student should be able to

- Define the responsibilities of the medical assistant.
- Name available sources of information about state laws.
- Describe how medical assisting in a small one-assistant office differs from assisting in a multiple-assistant office.
- Give the purpose of the health team.

The role and function of the medical assistant is constantly changing. The assistant is the doctor's helper and aide, the patient's friend and nurse, the other office employees' co-worker, and an office manager. In addition to these roles, the assistant is also a member of the community health team. A health team is made up of doctors, nurses, technicians, assistants, therapists, aides, and many others who work together in hospitals, clinics, planning agencies, environmental departments, and other types of groups to protect the health and well-being of members of the community. This team works together to maintain and restore good health to members of the community.

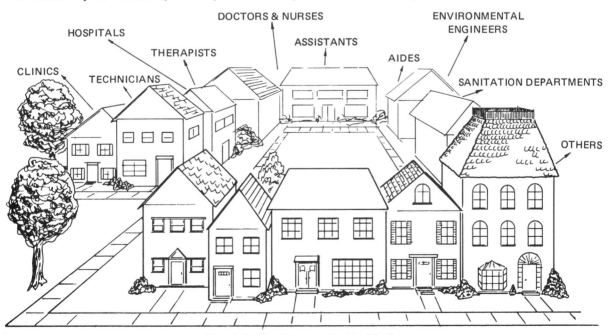

Fig. 1-1 The Community Health Team.

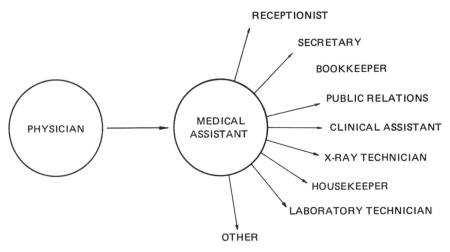

Fig. 1-2 **The one-assistant office.**

The duties of the medical assistant will vary greatly from office to office as well as from community to community. In a rural setting for example, the assistant may be the only help the doctor has in the office. This means that she will fill the role of medical assistant, clinician, receptionist, secretary, records keeper, bookkeeper, public relations manager, housekeeper, and office manager. It may be necessary to perform all the jobs and responsibilities that are required to run a doctor's office efficiently.

In a large city office where there are several people working for the doctor, each person will have a separate set of duties and each will fill a different role. In this situation, there may be one person responsible for each of the tasks the assistant in a small office is required to handle. In a large office or clinic, the doctor may have a laboratory technician, an x-ray technician, a medical secretary, a clinical assistant, a bookkeeper, a receptionist, and a housekeeper working for him. This means that the job skills demanded of an assistant will depend a great deal upon the size of the office as well as the size of the community. Another factor which influences the role of the assistant is the type of practice; some physicians are general practitioners and

some are specialists. The kind of practice that the physician is engaged in will naturally affect the types of duties an assistant will have.

RESPONSIBILITIES

The medical assistant's responsibilities are many. The assistant is responsible to:

- The doctor-employer for seeing that his office is well run and a professional, efficient atmosphere is maintained.

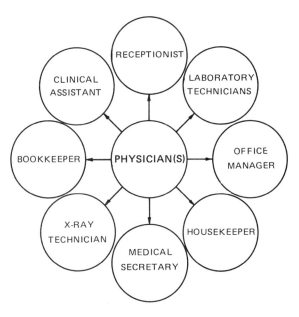

Fig. 1-3 **The multiple-assistant office.**

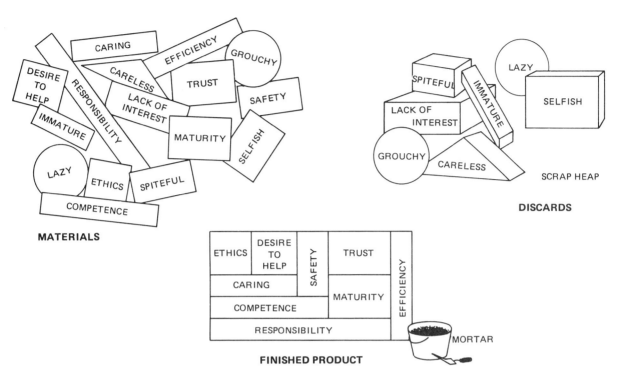

Fig. 1-4 Developing qualities of a good medical assistant.

- The patients for courteous, friendly, and competent care.

- Co-workers for harmony and cooperation in working together.

- Herself for maintaining high ideals and a sincere desire to serve others.

Unless the assistant recognizes and meets these responsibilities in a mature manner, the goal of becoming a successful member of the community health team will not be achieved.

A competent, mature, and responsible assistant will help the doctor by seeing that his office is run in an efficient and well-organized manner. This will save the doctor time and money and will benefit the patients by giving them the best care possible in the least amount of time. Good organization and efficiency will make the work much easier and more pleasant. Many of the specific duties of the assistant are covered in later chapters.

LAWS GOVERNING MEDICAL ASSISTING

The laws governing medical assisting are vitally important and *must be well known to the assistant for the assistant's own protection, the legal protection of the physician, and the safety of the patient.* State laws regulating medical practices and the workers in the medical field vary widely from state to state. Generally, the assistant is directly and legally responsible to the physician for all of her activities. In turn, the doctor is legally responsible to the patient for all activities that occur in his office relating to that patient's care. In some states, drug administration requires a license; permission by the physician is not enough. In time, all states will require that the assistant have a license before giving any medications. Laws will be passed which govern medical assisting and the duties performed, much like the nurse practice acts which control the practice of nursing. State laws should be carefully checked to determine the legal implications for the medical assistant. Contact the state medical association or the legislative body to obtain this information. Know the state laws governing medical assisting!

ETHICS

Ethics is a code of conduct and a standard of behavior based on high moral and professional principles and ideals. It is the practice of doing what is morally right at all times. The Golden Rule is a good principle of ethics and one that is especially important when dealing with people who are sick, unhappy, and frightened.

While no one is perfect, we can do our very best at all times. This means being honest, truthful, trustworthy, and responsible. It also means upholding the professional ethics of the field of medicine in dealing with patients, families, and other members of the health profession. Unethical people are a threat and a danger to the patients served and to the medical profession and must not be tolerated. Legal action involving lawsuits, fines, and sometimes imprisonment are frequently the results of unethical practices.

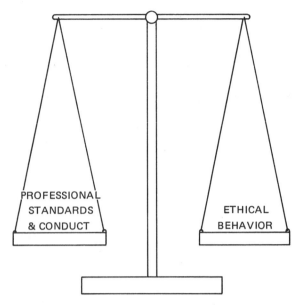

Fig. 1-5 Ethics of the medical assistant.

Therefore, it is necessary to learn the state laws governing medical assisting and to abide by them at all times. Patients and employers are entitled to receive treatment based on moral and ethical behavior in addition to legal principles. By following these guidelines for conduct and basing all activities on them, the medical assistant can function safely, efficiently, and competently as an important member of the health team.

SUGGESTED ACTIVITIES

Under the direction of your instructor, make arrangements to:

- Visit your family physician's office and observe his assistants at their duties. (This activity is best done on an individual basis. A group discussion can give an overall view of the different types of offices visited.)

- Have a lawyer speak to the group about state laws as they relate to the physician and his assistant. Include a question-and-answer session at the end of the lecture.

- Invite a medical assistant from a small office (one-assistant) to explain her duties and responsibilities to the group.

- Invite a medical assistant from a large clinic to discuss her duties and responsibilities. In a group discussion, compare the duties of this assistant with the duties of the assistant from a small (one-assistant) office.

REVIEW

A. Using a dictionary, define the following words.

role   legislation   profession
aspects   ethics   competence
moral

B. Answer the following questions.

1. List the responsibilities of the medical office assistant to:

    a. the physician

    b. the patients

    c. co-workers

    d. herself

2. In a small rural community, what roles would a medical assistant be expected to fill?

3. How do these responsibilities differ from those of an assistant in a multiple-assistant office?

4. Explain the meaning of ethics.

5. Name three factors which determine the job skills demanded of an assistant.

6. What is the purpose of the health team?

7. List three qualities which the medical assistant must have in order to help the doctor, and to operate the office efficiently.

8. Name one well-known ethical principle.

9. If an assistant made a mistake that injured a patient and the patient decided to sue for the injuries, who would be legally responsible for the injury of the patient?

10. Where can information be obtained concerning state laws that govern medical assisting?

11. Name three possible results of unethical practice.

Unit 2 The Patient

OBJECTIVES

After studying this unit, the student should be able to

- Describe reasons why a new patient may be fearful.
- Explain why good public relations is necessary.
- Give reasons why a medical history is of value to the patient, the physician, and the staff.

The patient and his esteem is of great importance to the conscientious assistant. The fears and anxieties a patient experiences play a major role in his behavior. The assistant must understand this and help the patient to cope with his feelings.

ESTABLISHING RAPPORT

Fear of the unknown is probably the greatest fear of man. A new situation will produce anxiety and fear to some degree. This anxiety is more obvious in some people than in others and must be coped with in individual ways. The medical assistant must learn to recognize this anxiety in its many forms and to help the patient cope with it. This should be done in a way that will put the patient at ease and relieve as much of his anxiety as possible.

If the patient is making his first visit to the office, he will probably have a higher level of anxiety than a returning patient. Meeting new people, being in a strange environment, fearing unknown and frightening procedures, and being concerned about his physical condition, frequently combine to make the patient very nervous and apprehensive. It is the assistant's duty to relieve these fears as much as possible. An atmosphere of genuine concern and sincerity for the patient should be created. The patient will feel better and be more cooperative in this type of atmosphere. The

duties of the assistant will also be easier. Establishing good *rapport* or a link of feeling and communication with the patient is an important first step in this direction. If the patient thinks that the assistant understands how he feels and is truly interested in him, then rapport has been established.

Whether the patient is new to the office or is returning, he must always be treated as an individual. Never should any patient be treated as just another medical case. All persons need recognition as individuals regardless of who or where they are; this is especially true in a physician's office where the patient is not feeling his best physically and is anxious and depressed mentally. The assistant must always be aware of this need and must always treat patients with dignity and respect.

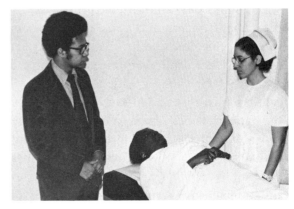

Fig. 2-1 Even though a patient may be glad to receive attention, fear of the unknown is present.

Patients often have fears and problems which require a sympathetic ear and an interested listener. The medical assistant should be able to demonstrate a professional, sincere interest in all patients.

PUBLIC RELATIONS

The patient's attitude toward the physician and his opinion of the physician and his staff can be greatly damaged or enhanced by one employee's attitudes and actions toward that patient. All employees of the doctor are a part of the public relations staff. Patients appreciate the kindness, consideration, empathy, and respect shown them by a thoughtful doctor and staff. If these qualities are not present, the patient will speedily take his ills elsewhere and frequently the bad publicity an office can receive is justly deserved.

Often office procedures become so familiar to the staff that they forget these same procedures are unknown and frightening to the patient. Every effort must be made to see that the patient understands what is being done to him and to answer any questions he may have about the procedure. This rule should always be followed regardless of the procedure. Be sure the patient understands what is being done and why it is being done, if at all possible. Never lie to a patient; do not minimize painful or uncomfortable procedures. If the patient understands what to expect and what is being done, he will be more cooperative and less fearful about an unfamiliar procedure. Being honest with the patient will gain his trust. The ability to "put yourself in the patient's shoes" can be a tremendous asset in dealing with frightened, insecure, or difficult patients. This will better enable the medical assistant to help the patients adjust to the new situation illness presents. The medical assistant is the patient's link between the familiar world and the unknown, frightening world of illness.

THE MEDICAL HISTORY

In some offices, the assistant will obtain the patient's medical history for the doctor. In other offices, the doctor will prefer to do this himself. In either case, there will be a printed form to follow in obtaining the desired information from the patient. The data will include general information about the family history such as the health of the parents, brothers, sisters, etc. and a personal medical history including any surgery, major illnesses, or injuries. If a patient refuses to answer any questions, do not pressure him; the doctor can obtain this information later. Occasionally men are reluctant to discuss their medical history with a female assistant.

The medical history is very important and becomes part of the patient's permanent personal file. All information must be recorded accurately. These records are legal documents and are subject to use as legal evidence in a court of law. Any information given to the physician or his staff is absolutely confidential and must be carefully protected. Information is never given out about any patient, and anything heard in a medical office is never to be discussed outside the office. Failure to observe this ethical and legal principle can result in legal action against the physician and his staff.

SUMMARY

A patient has fears and anxieties about himself and about being in a strange, unknown situation when he enters the doctor's office. It is the duty of the assistant to recognize and relieve those fears as much as possible and to make the patient feel more at ease by establishing good rapport with him.

Always tell the patient what is being done to him and why. Failure to do this may result in a frightened, uncooperative patient.

All information about a patient is confidential and must be protected. Office records are legal documents which may be used in a court of law and must be kept accurately and up-to-date.

Public relations are an important part of a medical office. A patient must feel that the doctor and his staff are genuinely interested in his welfare and will always treat him with respect and dignity. The patient is always an individual and must be treated as such.

SUGGESTED ACTIVITIES

- In a series of role-playing activities, a student plays the part of an assistant while a classmate plays the role of one of the following types of patients.

  a. A patient who is shy, frightened, and difficult to talk with.

  b. An extremely nervous, anxious, agitated patient.

  c. A frightened six-year-old who has never been a patient before.

  d. A gruff, uncooperative, reluctant, elderly man.

- Discuss the following situation from the patient's point of view.

  Mr. Jones has a four o'clock appointment. He arrives on time but is ignored by the assistant. Patiently he waits for fifteen minutes then approaches the assistant who is filing her nails. When asked how long it will be until the doctor can see him she responds with the statement that he must wait his turn. He returns to his seat and she returns to her nails for ten minutes more. The assistant then goes into the back of the office area for several minutes and returns with a nod for Mr. Jones to approach her desk. When he does so, she begins questioning him about his medical history in a loud, bored voice that is heard by all others in the waiting room. Finally, she tells him to "sit down" and she silently pops a thermometer into his mouth and begins to take his blood pressure which has never been checked before. When finished, she tells him to go back and sit down until he is called.

REVIEW

1. What is considered to be man's greatest fear?

2. What connection does this fear have with a patient who comes to see the doctor for the first time?

3. What is the legal importance of patient records?

4. What do you think a patient's feelings would be about returning to an office where he had been treated with dignity and respect?

5. How would a patient feel about an office where he had been treated with boredom and/or unconcern?

6. If the cousin of a patient calls on the telephone and wants to know what is wrong with the patient and just how sick he really is, what will you tell her?

7. Who is responsible for public relations in a doctor's office and why?

Unit 3 Vital Signs, Height and Weight

OBJECTIVES

After studying this unit, the student should be able to

- Define vital signs and list the equipment necessary to measure them.

- Measure and record temperature, pulse, respiration, blood pressure, height and weight.

- Give examples of situations where an oral temperature cannot be taken and indicate other ways in which the temperature could be taken.

Vital signs, or life signs, are important measurements of the body's state of health. These include temperature, pulse, respirations, and blood pressure. Height and weight are included in this because they are often all measured at the same time. Hands are washed thoroughly before and after each patient contact.

TEMPERATURE

Heat is produced by the body as it uses the food needed to maintain normal body functions. Food consumed through the alimentary canal is converted into a form that the body cells can oxidize; energy is then distributed to other parts of the body by the circulatory system. Heat is lost from the body by several means:

- perspiration
- respiration
- radiation
- convection
- saliva
- urine
- feces

The balance maintained by the production and loss of body heat is the normal body temperature. Body temperature is one of the vital signs. A sharp rise or drop in the temperature indicates there is a change from the body's normal condition. Normally, the temperature will vary slightly during a twenty-four hour cycle due to many factors other than illness. An abnormally high temperature is called a fever; the patient is febrile. Fever is not an illness but a symptom of a physical disorder.

The normal body temperature is usually considered in a range between 97.6°F (36.4°C) and 99.6°F (37.5°C). F stands for Fahrenheit which is one of the two common methods of measuring heat. Celsius (also called centigrade) is the other method; it is the metric system reading. The metric system of measurement is used in most countries of the world.

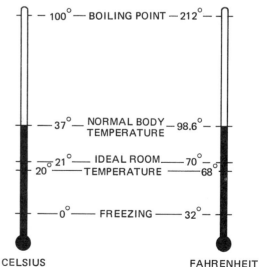

Fig. 3-1 Celsius and Fahrenheit Scales.

11

Thermometers are available with Fahrenheit or Celsius scales. Although the thermometer with the Fahrenheit scale has been extensively used and is still most popular, one should be aware of the trend to the metric system.

Body temperature is measured with two types of clinical thermometers. One is an oral thermometer which is a long, thin glass tube with a bulb at one end that is thin and longer than the other thermometer. Mercury is stored in this bulb and when heated expands upward through the glass tube which is calibrated in degrees and tenths of degrees. The rectal thermometer is very similar except that the bulb is shorter and fatter than that of the oral thermometer. Both types of thermometers are capable of registering temperature from 94°F (34.4°C) to 107°F (41.7°C).

Three methods of measuring temperature are used. An oral temperature can be taken by placing an oral thermometer underneath the tongue with the lips firmly closed for 3 to 5 minutes. The patient should have had no hot or cold substances in his mouth for at least 15 minutes. After 3 to 5 minutes, the thermometer is removed from the mouth, wiped with a clean, soft tissue from the hand toward the bulb, read, and cleaned.

A rectal temperature is taken by gently placing a well-lubricated rectal thermometer about one inch into the rectum and leaving it for 3 to 5 minutes. The best lubricants for rectal thermometers are water-soluble which dissipate rapidly, such as petroleum jelly. The thermometer is then carefully removed, wiped in the same manner, read, and cleaned. The rectal temperature is the most accurate measurement of body temperature and will register about one full degree higher (99.6°F or 37.5°C) than an oral temperature.

An axillary temperature is taken with a clinical thermometer by placing the thermometer under the axilla or armpit for at least 10 minutes. The axilla should be dry and the

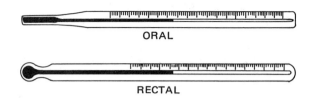

Fig. 3-2 Clinical thermometer. Note the tips of the thermometers.

thermometer placed so that it does not rest in an air pocket. The patient's arm should be held firmly at his side to hold the thermometer in place. This method is used only when it is not possible to take a temperature orally or rectally. This is the least accurate of all methods. The axillary temperature will usually register at least one full degree below the oral reading. It is charted as Ax. 97.6° if a Fahrenheit thermometer is used (36.4° Celsius or Centigrade).

To prepare to measure temperature, a clean clinical thermometer is removed from its container, read, and carefully shaken down by holding it tightly between the thumb and first two fingers. A quick, downward shake of the wrist will force the mercury into the bulb. This procedure must be repeated until the thermometer registers 96°F or below. To read a thermometer, hold it horizontally by the glass end at eye level. Slowly rotate the thermometer with the fingers until the dark line made by the mercury can be seen in the center of the thermometer. The end of the mercury line is the temperature measurement.

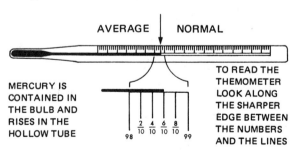

Fig. 3-3 Reading a clinical thermometer.

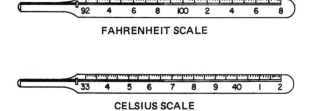

FAHRENHEIT SCALE

CELSIUS SCALE

Fig. 3-4 Thermometers are available in the Fahrenheit and Celsius scales.

Be very careful in shaking down a thermometer; the thermometer is made of glass and if hit upon anything will shatter and spill mercury, which is a dangerous element. Should a patient ever break a thermometer in his mouth, have him rinse his mouth immediately and notify the doctor. Also, never put a thermometer into hot water since the mercury will expand to the point that the thermometer is no longer usable.

Always explain to the patient that you are going to take his temperature. If for any reason, the patient cannot hold a thermometer in his mouth safely, take the temperature by rectum or axilla. Oral temperatures must not be taken in the following cases;

- unconscious, convulsive, delirous, or mentally disturbed patients.

- patients with mouth injuries or breathing problems who cannot keep their lips closed tightly long enough for the temperature to register.

- infants or children who are not old enough to understand how to hold a thermometer properly in their mouths.

After using a thermometer it should be correctly cleaned by washing it carefully in cold soapy water and rinsing it well in cold, running water. After drying with a soft, clean tissue, the thermometer is placed in a disinfectant solution of 70% alcohol and left to soak for at least 10 minutes. It is then removed, rinsed again in cold, running water, wiped dry

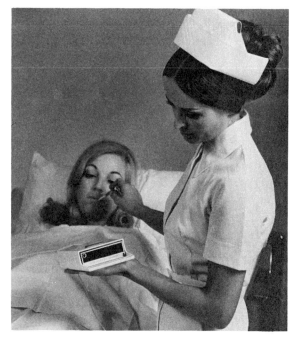

Fig. 3-5 Using an electronic thermometer.

and stored in a clean container with a top. The bulb of the thermometer should rest on clean, soft cotton.

NOTE: Always rinse a thermometer well to remove all traces of alcohol before placing it into the patient's mouth or rectum.

The electronic thermometer is replacing the regular thermometers in some offices and hospitals.

PULSE

When the heart contracts (beats) it forces blood throughout the body by way of the blood vessels. This contraction or heartbeat can be measured in pulsations per minute by placing the index finger over an artery that lies between the surface of the skin and a hard surface beneath the vessel, such as a bone. The pressure felt by the fingertip is constantly changing from more to less in a regular, rhythmic beat that can be counted; this is the *pulse*. It can be felt at the radial or brachial artery.

The *radial artery* is the artery most commonly used for counting the pulse. It is found

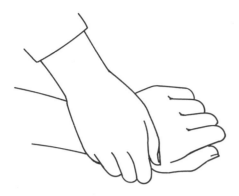

Fig. 3-6 Finding the radial pulse.

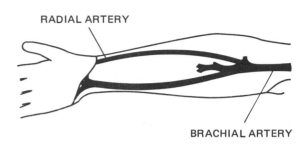

Fig. 3-7 The radial and brachial arteries.

on the inside of the wrist above the thumbs of either hand. Gentle pressure with the index finger against the bones of the arm will help locate the pulse. Never use the thumb directly on the inside wrist or you will be counting your own pulse. After locating the pulse, count it for one full minute using a watch with a second hand. To count accurately takes a great amount of practice. Accuracy is absolutely necessary!

Before counting a pulse, inform the patient of your intentions. Place the patient in a comfortable position. To check the patient's pulse it is best to place the patient's arm across his chest while he is lying on his back. (In this way the patient's respirations can be counted without his knowledge; he will believe that his pulse is still being counted.) When the patient is comfortable, find the radial pulse and count it for a full minute. Until the medical assistant is proficient at this procedure, the pulse should always be counted for a minute, twice to be sure of an accurate count.   After confidence and skill through practice is obtained, pulse count may be taken for 30 seconds and multiplied by two. Write the pulse down immediately before it is forgotten. The pulse and respiration are usually counted while the temperature is being taken, that is, the thermometer is in the patient's mouth. This saves time and also prevents the patient from talking and interrupting the counting process.

An abnormally fast pulse rate is called *tachycardia* and indicates that the heart is racing. An abnormally slow pulse rate is called *bradycardia* and indicates that the heart is pumping below the normal rate.

Average Normal Pulse Rate	
Age	**Beats per Minute**
Men	60-70
Women	70-80
1 to 7 year old child	80-120
Child over 7 years old	80-90
Newborn babies	130-160
Infants	110-130

RESPIRATION

Respiration is one full cycle of breathing in (called *inhalation*) and breathing out (called *exhalation*). Oxygen is inhaled with the air and carbon dioxide and other gases are exhaled from the body. The oxygen is absorbed by the lungs and circulated throughout the body to all the cells by the circulatory system. This same system picks up carbon dioxide and other waste products that are eliminated from the body. The carbon dioxide leaves the body by way of the lungs.

Counting the patient's respiration should always be done without his knowledge since respiration can be controlled by the patient.

Being aware that someone is watching will alter one's breathing rate. As previously indicated, the best time to count respiration is when checking the pulse, either before or after. By placing the patient's arm across his chest while taking his pulse, the respiration count can also be taken; this is done by feeling the rise and fall of the chest. However, sometimes patients find this uncomfortable. If the pulse is taken with the arm placed elsewhere, the medical assistant must be sure she can watch the chest movements and count them without the patient being aware of it.

Count the respirations for one full minute. Note the type of respiration, such as regular or irregular. Also note the quality of respiration, such as difficult, wheezy, shallow, or other description. Write down the number of respirations as soon as the count is completed.

Several factors which affect the respiration count are exercise immediately before counting, anxiety, nervousness, pain, or congestion.

Report any unusual observations to the doctor as soon as possible and record the information on the record.

Normal Respiratory Rates for One Minute	
Men	14-18
Women	18-20
Children	20-26
Infants	30-38

BLOOD PRESSURE

The pressure the blood exerts on the walls of blood vessels as it is pumped out to the heart and through the circulatory system is called *blood pressure.* As the heart contracts, blood is forced out of the heart and into the arteries that carry it to all parts of the body. This force causes the pressure inside the arteries to increase and this stage of the cardiac cycle is called *systole* or the contraction stage.

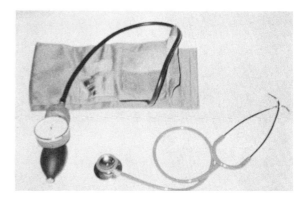

Fig. 3-8 Aneroid sphygmomanometer and stethoscope.

In the second stage of the cardiac cycle, the the pressure decreases inside the arteries and this stage is called *diastole* or relaxation stage. The systolic pressure will be greater than the diastolic pressure.

Blood pressure is the actual measurement of the systolic pressure (always written as the numerator of a fraction) and the diastolic pressure (written as the denominator of a fraction). For example: $\frac{130}{80}$. The systolic rate is 130 and the diastolic rate is 80. Blood pressure is an indicator of the general health of the body. Many factors will affect blood pressure such as age, sex, emotional state, exercise, and weight. An abnormally high blood pressure is a condition known as *hypertension.* An abnormally low blood pressure is *hypotension.*

The equipment necessary for measuring blood pressure is a *sphygmomanometer* (sphyg-mo-man-om-eter). This apparatus consists of a cuff that wraps around the patient's arm about one inch above the elbow, a rubber bulb (attached to the cuff by a rubber tube) and a measuring device called a manometer; this manometer is also attached to the cuff. One type of manometer is called an *aneroid* manometer which consists of a metal bellows that causes a needle to move across a round, glass, calibrated dial, figure 3-8. The other type of manometer is called a *mercury* manometer which is a column containing mercury and is marked in millimeters, figure 3-9.

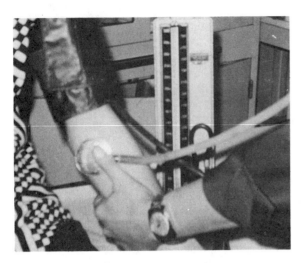

Fig. 3-9 Taking a blood pressure with a mercury gravity manometer.

The other piece of equipment necessary to take a blood pressure is a *stethoscope*. This is a device for listening to the sounds transmitted from the area where the blood pressure is being checked (brachial artery). A bell-like or medallion device is placed over the brachial artery; rubber tubing transmits the sounds to two earpieces that fit into the listener's ears. The sound transmitted is a thump-thump, thump-thump sound. The stethoscope is used with both kinds of manometers.

When taking a blood pressure, explain the procedure to the patient and have him sit or lie down in a comfortable position. The left arm is usually used and should be at the same level as the heart. The brachial artery is found on the inside of the elbow near the body. When the arm is extended, inside of elbow up, the artery can be located by using the same method as used for checking a pulse. The stethoscope bell should be placed directly over the brachial artery.

The cuff is wrapped securely around the patient's arm about one inch above the elbow and fastened. Air is pumped into the cuff by closing the small valve beside the bulb and then squeezing the bulb until the manometer reads about 180. (This is done to avoid pumping to

an unnecessary, high, uncomfortable point.) Stop pumping and listen for a thumping sound. If a thumping sound *is* heard, continue pumping until the manometer reads about 200. When no thumping sound is heard, slowly release the air valve beside the bulb; the manometer reading will drop as air escapes from the cuff. Listen carefully! The number indicated on the manometer when the *first thumping sound* is heard is the *systolic* pressure. For example: The systolic pressure may be 130. Remember this number! Continue to let the air escape and the pressure fall slowly until the continuous thumping sound stops. The point on the manometer where the sound is very difficult to hear or *stops* is the reading for the *diastolic* pressure. For example: The diastolic pressure may reach 80. Remember it! Let the remainder of the air out of the cuff and allow the patient to flex his arm. Write down the systolic and diastolic reading. Take the blood pressure a second time to be sure your first reading was accurate. Follow the same procedure. The medical assistant must practice this procedure until there are no errors. The blood pressure should be taken quickly as the pressure of the cuff can cause the patient discomfort. After its use, clean the equipment by wiping the bell and earpieces of the stethoscope with an alcohol sponge. Return all equipment to its proper place.

Record all vital signs as follows:

    T.   98.6°

    P.   76

    R.   14

    B.P. $\frac{130}{80}$

HEIGHT AND WEIGHT

Height and weight are often measured at the same time the vital signs are measured. This is a simple procedure and usually accomplished with standard upright scales. If possible have the patient dressed in an examination

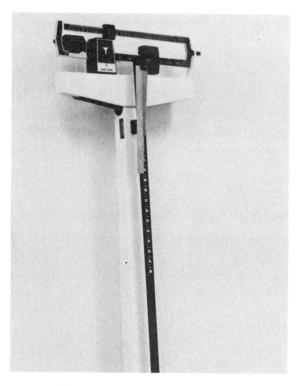

Fig. 3-10 Standard upright scales.

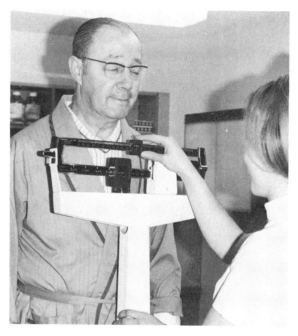

Fig. 3-11 Measuring a patient's weight.

gown; shoes should be removed for accuracy, especially when measuring height. Place protective paper toweling on the scale if the patient is barefoot. Assist the patient onto the scales, balance them, note and record the weight. While the patient is still on the scales, measure his height. Have the patient stand erect and lower the height lever until it rests lightly upon the top of the patient's head. Note and record the reading. The reading should be recorded in feet, inches, and fractions of inches. Assist the patient off the scales.

SUMMARY

Vital signs, or signs of life, are essential in determining the state of a person's health; they include temperature, pulse, respiration, and blood pressure. Usually the height and weight are recorded at the time the vital signs are taken. All readings and measurements must be absolutely accurate and recorded without error. These procedures may require much practice in order to do them with ease, skill and accuracy. All safety precautions must be observed. The patient must always be told beforehand about the procedures except counting respirations. Respirations may be altered if one is aware they are being counted.

SUGGESTED ACTIVITIES

- Review the circulatory system.

- Review the respiratory system.

- Practice measuring and charting the vital signs of classmates.

- Record the height and weight of classmates.

- Each student selects one or more of the following terms and gives a brief report on its meaning to the class. *All* terms must be discussed.

afebrile	dyspnea	orthopnea
apnea	hyperpnea	stertorous
bradycardia	hypertension	stridor
cyanosis	hypotension	tachycardia

REVIEW

A. Briefly answer the following questions.

1. Explain how body cells, the alimentary canal and the circulatory system produce body heat.

2. In the following list, encircle the vital signs.

cardiac cycle	pulse
temperature	weight
height	respirations
blood pressure	alimentary canal

3. a. What device is used to measure body heat?

   b. In what system is it calibrated at the present time?

   c. In terms of degrees, what are the actual measurements marked off on the thermometer?

4. List the three common methods of measuring body temperature, give their normal values, and tell how long the thermometer must be left in place to get an accurate reading.

5. Name two types of clinical thermometers and describe how they differ from each other.

6. List three types of cases when an oral temperature must not be taken.

7. a. Name a solution used to disinfect clinical thermometers.

   b. How long must the thermometers be left soaking in the solution?

8. a. Name the artery most commonly used for counting the pulse.

   b. Where is it located?

9. a. What artery is the one most often used for checking the blood pressure?

   b. Where is it located?

10. Why is the medical assistant's thumb never placed over the artery to count a pulse?

11. Name the stages which make up one full cycle of respiration.

12. Why should the respiratory rate be counted without the patient's knowledge?

13. Name and explain what happens during the two stages of the cardiac cycle.

14. a. Which stage of the cardiac cycle is associated with the systolic pressure?

    b. Which stage of the cardiac cycle is associated with diastolic pressure?

15. Name the two instruments which make up a blood pressure kit.

16. Name the gases inhaled and exhaled during respiration.

17. Name the two types of manometers and give a brief description of each.

18. Why is cold water used to clean thermometers?

19. Why are the T.P.R. and B.P. called vital signs?

20. a. What is an abnormally fast pulse rate called?

    b. What is an abnormally slow pulse rate called?

21. a. What is another term for high blood pressure?

    b. What term may describe low blood pressure?

B. Complete the following items.

1. Pulse rate is actually an indication of the number of _____ per minute.

2. The blood pressure is an indicator of the _____ _____ .

3. The beginning of a thumping sound when taking a blood pressure is the _____ phase and the cessation of the sound is the _____ phase.

4. The normal respiration rate for children is from _____ to _____ respirations per minute.

Unit 4 Charting

OBJECTIVES

After studying this unit, the student should be able to

- Give reasons why accurate medical records are important.

- List the rules for charting.

- Identify and demonstrate commonly used abbreviations, signs, and symbols in charting.

- Accurately and efficiently chart specific information on medical records.

The records maintained in a doctor's office are vitally important. In addition to having legal implications, these records are an accurate, running account of the patient's health, illness, injuries, diagnostic procedures, treatments, and progress. All records must be

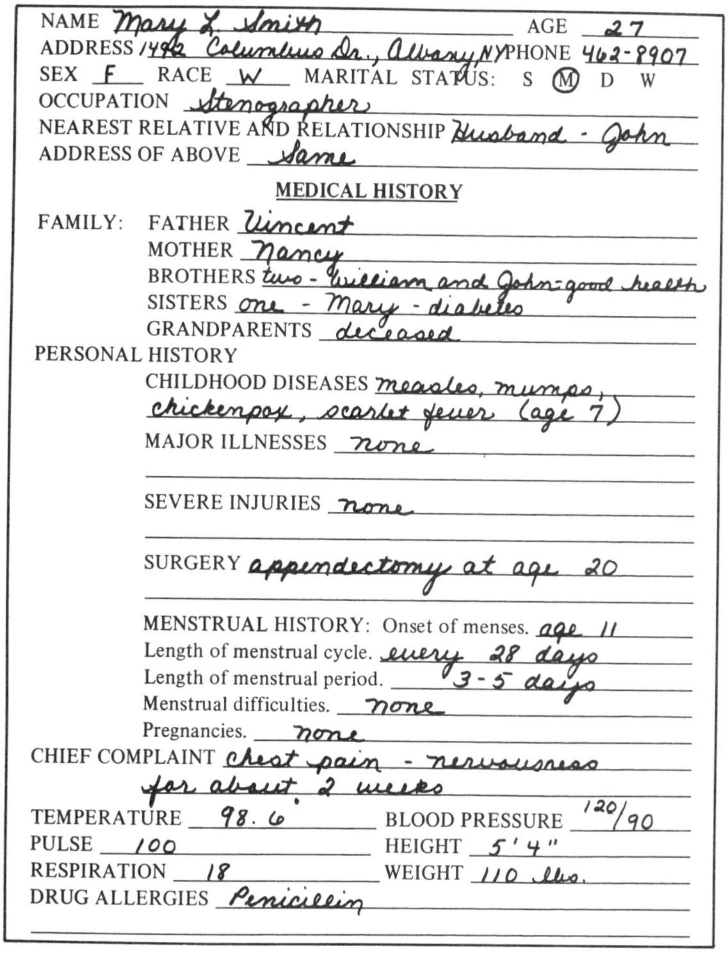

NAME *Mary L. Smith* AGE *27*
ADDRESS *1442 Columbus Dr., Albany, NY* PHONE *462-8907*
SEX *F* RACE *W* MARITAL STATUS: S (M) D W
OCCUPATION *Stenographer*
NEAREST RELATIVE AND RELATIONSHIP *Husband - John*
ADDRESS OF ABOVE *Same*

MEDICAL HISTORY

FAMILY: FATHER *Vincent*
    MOTHER *Nancy*
    BROTHERS *two - William and John - good health*
    SISTERS *one - Mary - diabetes*
    GRANDPARENTS *deceased*
PERSONAL HISTORY
    CHILDHOOD DISEASES *measles, mumps, chickenpox, scarlet fever (age 7)*
    MAJOR ILLNESSES *none*

    SEVERE INJURIES *none*

    SURGERY *appendectomy at age 20*

    MENSTRUAL HISTORY: Onset of menses. *age 11*
    Length of menstrual cycle. *every 28 days*
    Length of menstrual period. *3-5 days*
    Menstrual difficulties. *none*
    Pregnancies. *none*
CHIEF COMPLAINT *chest pain - nervousness for about 2 weeks*
TEMPERATURE *98.6°* BLOOD PRESSURE *120/90*
PULSE *100* HEIGHT *5'4"*
RESPIRATION *18* WEIGHT *110 lbs.*
DRUG ALLERGIES *Penicillin*

Fig. 4-1 A medical history.

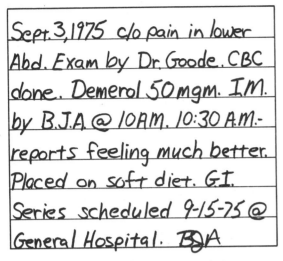

Fig. 4-2 A. Correct charting technique.

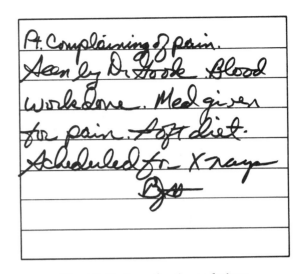

Fig. 4-2 B. Poor charting technique.

accurate, legible, and kept up-to-date. The medical history must be informative and accurate.

Records are useless unless they serve their intended purpose. They must be clear, factual and legible accounts of the patient's health and the care he receives in the doctor's office. Records must be neat, accurate, and concise. Each office will vary somewhat in its method of record keeping but each method will conform to the general rules of charting or record keeping.

GENERAL RULES FOR CHARTING

- Be certain that the information being charted is recorded about the right patient and on the correct form. Check the name on the record when it is pulled from the file and again before charting.

- All information must be written in a clear, legible manner. Charted material is usually printed as printing is easier to read. All charting is done in ink — never pencil.

- Whenever an entry is made on any record, the person recording the entry must sign or initial the entry. The month, day, and the year must precede all entries.

- All diagnostic procedures, treatments, medications, and the results (including unexpected reactions, if any) are carefully recorded. Any information about the patient is entered on his particular record.

- All unusual complaints, symptoms, or reactions are noted in detail. Also, the assistant must learn to be very observant and to record anything that seems to be pertinent to the care of the patient.

- The spelling, abbreviations, symbols, and terminology used must always be correct.

USE OF MEDICAL TERMINOLOGY

Medical terminology differs greatly from the ordinary language. An approved medical dictionary is an invaluable and necessary tool in maintaining medical records. There are several publications available which will provide practice. However, since medical terms are changing and constantly increasing, it is up to the assistant to learn each new word when it is heard and read. Whenever an unfamiliar word is encountered, the medical assistant must learn its meaning, learn to spell it correctly, and learn how it is used in medical

@	at		I.V.	intravenous
a̅a̅	of each		lb.	pound
abd.	abdomen		liq.	liquid
amb.	ambulatory (able to walk)		mg	milligram
amt.	amount		ml	milliliter
Ax.	axillary		mm	millimeter
BP	blood pressure		N & V	nausea and vomiting
C.	Celsius (centigrade)		noc.	at night
c̅	with		NPO	nothing by mouth
CBC	complete blood count		OB	obstetrics
cc	cubic centimeter		o.d.	right eye
CC	chief complaint (in medical history)		OOB	out of bed
dil.	dilute		o.s.	left eye
disc.	discontinue		p.o.	by mouth
EENT	eye, ear, nose, and throat		PRN	as necessary
elix.	elixir		q.d.	every day
ENT	ear, nose, and throat		q.o.d.	every other day
F.	Fahrenheit		R.	rectal
Fx	fracture		℞	prescription
GI	gastrointestinal		RBC	red blood cell
GU	genitourinary		s̅	without
GYN	gynecology		s.c. or sub. cu.	subcutaneous
Hb or Hgb	hemoglobin		sol.	solution
H'crit or Hct	hematocrit		sp. gr.	specific gravity
Ht.	height		TPR	temperature, pulse, and respiration
I.M.	intramuscular		WBC	white blood cell
			W/C	wheel chair
			wt.	weight

Fig. 4-3 Frequently used abbreviations.

language. A composition notebook is useful for listing new medical terms and their definitions.

Learning medical terminology is an ongoing process of vocabulary growth. Constant reference to a good medical dictionary is an essential element of this growth in knowledge. The medical assistant is responsible for increasing her own knowledge by making each new medical term a working part of her medical vocabulary.

ABBREVIATIONS USED IN CHARTING

There are many abbreviations used in recording and charting. These abbreviations, signs, and symbols will vary in usage in different geographical areas. It will be necessary for the medical assistant to become familiar with abbreviations used in her particular area and office. A few commonly used abbreviations are shown in figure 4-3. The medical dictionary is an excellent reference for additional abbreviations.

SUMMARY

Good charting and recording must be clear, concise, accurate, and legible. All entries should be carefully printed in ink on the patient's record. Accurate spelling and use of correct terminology is vitally important. Remember the rules for proper recording of data and BE ACCURATE!

SUGGESTED ACTIVITIES

- Using a medical dictionary, define the following words.

anatomy	leukemia
biopsy	malignant
cardiac	nocturnal
catheter	occlusion
diuretic	palpation
exudate	prognosis
foramen	trauma

- Using the form below, obtain the necessary information from a classmate acting as the patient; and record it properly.

NAME _____ AGE _____

ADDRESS _____ PHONE _____

SEX _____ RACE _____ MARITAL STATUS: S M D W

OCCUPATION _____

NEAREST RELATIVE AND RELATIONSHIP _____

ADDRESS OF ABOVE _____

MEDICAL HISTORY

FAMILY: FATHER _____

MOTHER _____

BROTHERS _____

SISTERS _____

GRANDPARENTS _____

PERSONAL HISTORY

CHILDHOOD DISEASES _____

_____

MAJOR ILLNESSES _____

_____

SEVERE INJURIES _____

_____

SURGERY _____

_____

MENSTRUAL HISTORY: Onset of menses. _____

Length of menstrual cycle. _____

Length of menstrual period. _____

Menstrual difficulties. _____

Pregnancies. _____

CHIEF COMPLAINT _____

_____

TEMPERATURE _____ BLOOD PRESSURE _____

PULSE _____ HEIGHT _____

RESPIRATION _____ WEIGHT _____

DRUG ALLERGIES _____

REVIEW

A. Write the correct abbreviations for the following terms.

1. milligram _____
2. as necessary _____
3. at night _____
4. pound _____
5. intramuscular _____
6. amount _____
7. right eye _____
8. left eye _____
9. rectal _____
10. axillary _____

11. with _____
12. without _____
13. every other day _____
14. gastrointestinal _____
15. ear, nose, and throat _____
16. hematocrit _____
17. hemoglobin _____
18. ambulatory _____
19. of each _____

B. Chart the following information, using abbreviations when necessary.

1. Chief Complaint: Abdominal pain at night with occasional nausea and vomiting.
2. Rectal temperature: ninety nine and four-tenths degrees Fahrenheit.
3. Pulse: eighty six.
4. Height: five feet, four and one-third inches.
5. Weight: one hundred twenty-seven pounds.
6. Blood pressure: systolic — one hundred forty; diastolic — seventy.

C. Answer the questions briefly.

1. Why is printing rather than writing used on medical records?

2. What should the medical office assistant do when she encounters a word that is unfamiliar?

3. In addition to the date which precedes all entries on a record, what identifying factor is entered?

Unit 5 Preparation for the Physical Examination

OBJECTIVES

After studying this unit, the student should be able to

- Prepare the examination room, equipment, instruments, supplies, and other items for the examination.
- List the examination positions, identify them, and correctly demonstrate how to position and drape a patient.
- State and use guidelines to prepare the patient both emotionally and physically for examination.

The medical assistant must know how to prepare and use the examination room equipment and supplies needed for an examination. The medical assistant must also become proficient in preparing the patient for an examination. This unit will introduce the basic concepts necessary to the patient's comfort and the assistant's ease in this most important aspect of medical assisting.

PREPARATION OF THE EXAMINING ROOM

The examining room must be prepared for each procedure that is to be performed in it. This preparation will depend upon the type of procedure to be done. However, there are some general principles that apply to preparing for any kind of procedure.

Since an examining room must always be thoroughly cleaned after each use, it will be ready to set up for the examination procedure. The room should be maintained at a comfortable temperature and be well ventilated. Rooms that are kept at a comfortable temperature for working personnel may be too cold for a patient who must remove his clothing for the physical examination. If the room is cool, a light cotton blanket should be used to keep the patient warm until the examination begins.

Odors associated with illness and disease can be very upsetting to a person who is seeking medical care. Often these odors are familiar to the staff and, even though unpleasant, they are an accepted part of the job. Care should be taken not to expose patients to any unpleasant odors. Use good ventilation and a room deodorizer.

EQUIPMENT AND SUPPLIES

The examining room will contain an examination table made so that it can be adjusted according to the type of examination or treatment that is to be done, figure 5-2. The assistant must learn to adjust and manipulate

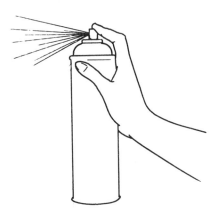

Fig. 5-1 Use of a deodorizer eliminates offensive odors.

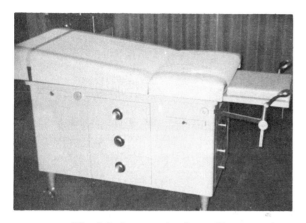

Fig. 5-2 An examination table.

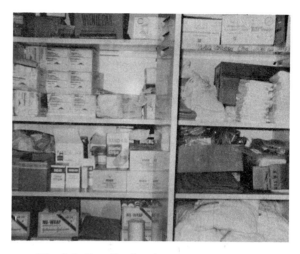

Fig. 5-3 Supplies for the examination room.

this equipment. The table must be covered with a clean sheet of cloth or paper which is mounted on a roll under one end of the table. The paper is pulled off the roll as needed. The used sheet is discarded after each patient. Paper sheeting is more commonly used as it is easy and considered to be more economical.

A stool is used by some physicians and must be placed in a convenient position. Care must be taken not to put it where staff or patients might trip over it. The same rule applies to footstools. With some examination tables, a stool must be used by the patient to reach the table. The newer examination tables have a platform that is stored in the table.

The examining room will contain cabinets with instruments, equipment, and supplies. The assistant must select the equipment which will be used by the physician and arrange the equipment on a clean tray that is covered with a clean hand towel. After the examination tray is set up with items that the doctor will need, it is covered with another clean towel and placed near the examination table within easy reach of the physician. The equipment will vary depending on the kind of examination the physician will be doing. Always check with the doctor to be sure all items he will need are provided. Specific examination and diagnostic procedures will be covered in a later unit.

PREPARING THE PATIENT

The patient must be prepared physically and emotionally. First, he must be informed of the examination so that he will know what to expect. The physician usually does this; however, the assistant may be responsible for this task. She will tell the patient what clothing must be removed and take the patient to an area or dressing room where this can be done in privacy. A sheet is given to the patient for cover when leaving the dressing area. Never leave a patient alone who is not feeling well enough to stand or move about. If the patient is unable to remove his or her own clothing, the assistant must help without causing any embarrassment. This is best done in a professional but helpful manner; the assistant should be considerate of the patients modesty and, yet, show no embarrassment. If the examination is to take place in another room, the assistant walks with the patient to the room. The examining room will be clean and ready for the patient.

Care is always taken not to expose a patient. Modesty should be respected and protected as much as possible. As soon as the patient is positioned on the table, the sheet is draped or arranged so that the patient is covered except for the area to be examined. The

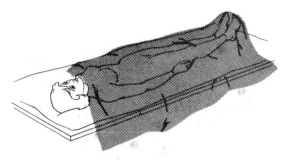

Fig. 5-4 The horizontal recumbent position.

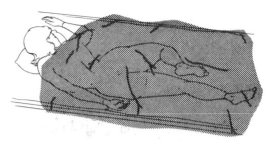

Fig. 5-5 Sims' position.

area to be examined should be temporarily covered with a towel or part of the draping until the doctor is ready to examine it.

An examination of any kind is often frightening and embarrassing to many people. The assistant should always be aware of this and be sensitive to the patient's feelings. By being considerate and thoughtful the assistant can make an examination less stressful for the patients.

Remember, if a patient understands the procedure to be done and knows that the medical assistant is considerate, he will be much more cooperative. Keep in mind that medical language used between members of the staff is not always appropriate in explaining procedures to a patient. Information must be given in a way the patient can understand. This does not mean talking to patients as if they were children, but speaking in understandable language, using nontechnical terms. Patients should be given the opportunity to ask questions about procedures they do not understand.

EXAMINATION POSITIONS

There are standard positions used for examinations and treatments. The position of the patient will depend upon what type of examination is to be done. The assistant will prepare the patient for examination by placing him in the correct position on the examination table and draping him with a sheet. Modesty is to be considered and preserved at all times. Some of the standard positions follow.

Horizontal Recumbent Position

This position is often referred to as *supine*, figure 5-4. In this position, the patient lies flat on the back in a comfortable position. A pillow may be placed under the head to make the position more comfortable. The arms may be crossed over the chest or allowed to rest at the sides. The legs are extended but not crossed. A sheet is loosely placed over the patient.

Lateral Position

This position is also called Sims' position, figure 5-5. The patient is placed on the left side with the left arm and shoulder front-side down on the table. This puts the body weight on the chest. The right arm is flexed, palm down, at a comfortable angle. The right leg is flexed at a 90° angle to the length of the body with the knee bent. The left leg is fairly straight (extended). The patient is draped with a sheet so that the buttocks or rectal area may be examined without uncovering the patient. If the patient desires, a small pillow may be placed underneath the head.

Prone Position

The patient lies on the abdomen in a flat position, figure 5-6. The head is turned in either direction, right or left. The arms may be flexed so the head can rest on the hands, or the hands can be extended at the sides. The patient is draped with a sheet from shoulders to feet.

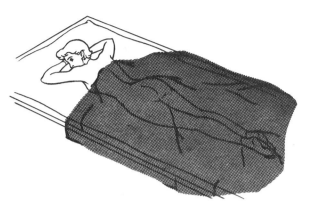

Fig. 5-6 The prone position.

Dorsal Recumbent Position

This position is sometimes referred to as the stirrup position, figure 5-7. It is most frequently used for vaginal or rectal examinations. The patient lies on the back covered with a sheet and moves to the lower edge of the examination table until the buttocks are near the edge. The medical asssitant will place each foot into a stirrup by supporting the patient's leg with both hands and placing the foot into a stirrup. The stirrups are extended about 18 to 20 inches above the level of the buttocks and should be about two feet apart. This is far enough away from the patient to keep the knees bent but not be uncomfortable. The sheet is draped to cover the body completely. The two corners near the feet are draped around the legs and feet and tucked into the stirrups. When the doctor begins the examination, the center of the lower edge of the sheet is raised and draped up over the patient's abdomen.

Jackknife and Knee-Chest Positions

The jackknife position is used for rectal or proctological examinations, figure 5-8. It is uncomfortable and the patient should not be positioned until the doctor is ready to examine the patient. The table must be positioned so that the patient can lie face down with the

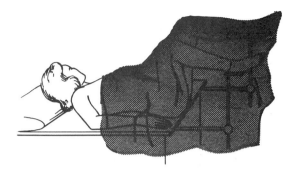

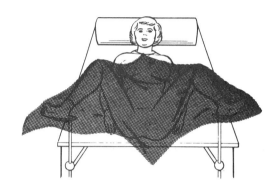

Fig. 5-7 Two views of the dorsal recumbent position. Note draping.

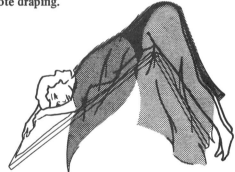

Fig. 5-8 The jackknife position.

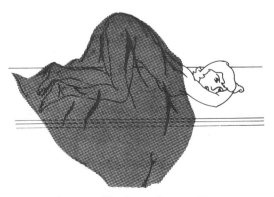

Fig. 5-9 The knee-chest position.

head and chest in a straight line with the buttocks the highest point. The head is lower than the buttocks. The legs form another straight line from the buttocks downward toward the feet. Two sheets are used in draping since the legs are slightly separated for the examination. One sheet covers the upper part of the body and one leg; the other sheet is used to cover the other leg. The patient must be carefully assisted into this position, supported well while in it, and helped out of it.

Many physicians will use the knee-chest position for rectal examinations, see figure 5-9. Notice the draping of the patient.

Sitting Position

In the sitting position, the patient faces the physician and sits in an upright position on the side of the examining table or at the foot of the table. The back is straight and the feet should rest on a stool or platform which extends from the table. A sheet is draped around the patient so that the physician can lower the sheet to examine the chest or back. It is usually placed around the patient under the arms so it can be held securely until the examination begins.

OTHER RESPONSIBILITIES OF THE ASSISTANT

The medical assistant will remain in the examining room to assist the physician unless she is requested not to stay. Men often are uncomfortable with a female assistant present during an examination. However, the assistant is always present during any treatment or examination of a female patient. This is for the emotional support of the patient and the protection of the physician against unscrupulous or untrue charges of misconduct.

When an examination is completed, the medical assistant helps the patient from the table, helps him to dress, if necessary, and escorts him to the physician's office for consultation with the doctor. After the patient has left the examination room, the supplies, instruments, and equipment must be cleaned and returned to their proper place by the medical assistant. Dirty linen goes into a hamper, instruments are washed in a solution of warm, soapy water, rinsed, and sterilized. Cleaned equipment is returned to its place and supplies are replaced if necessary. A disinfectant solution is used to wipe down the examining table and a clean piece of paper sheeting is put into place. If the pillow was used, the case must be replaced.

After each patient use, the examination or treatment room must always be cleaned and readied for the next patient. This will leave the room in condition for another patient or an emergency situation. *Hands are washed thoroughly and dried before and after each patient and each procedure.* Inventory is checked daily to maintain supplies.

SUMMARY

The assistant orders and maintains all supplies, equipment, and instruments in the examination or treatment rooms. She assists patients into correct examination positions and drapes them in a way that the doctor can perform the examination without exposing the patient unnecessarily. The medical assistant remains in the room at all times when the physician is with a female patient and assists with examinations of males unless instructed that it is not necessary. When the examination is completed, the patient is assisted from the examination table and helped to dress if such help is necessary. The medical assistant will clean all items used, replace supplies if needed, and leave the room ready for the next patient.

SUGGESTED ACTIVITIES

- Decide what positions would be used for the following examinations.
  - eye, ear, nose, and throat (EENT exam)
  - examination of spine
  - examination of the heart and lungs
  - pelvic examination
  - abdominal examination
- Practice positioning and draping procedures, using classmates as patients.
- In small groups, discuss how patients might feel about examinations and treatments in a doctor's office. Relate how past personal experiences in physicians' offices can be used to make each class member a better medical office assistant.

REVIEW

A. Briefly answer the following questions.

  1. Why is it necessary for the patient to understand what is to be done?

  2. How can the medical assistant help the patient who is about to have a physical examination?

  3. What are two things that should be considered in the examination room regarding the patient's comfort?

  4. What are two reasons that a female patient is never left unattended with the physician?

  5. When are the examination and treatment rooms checked for inventory, and supplies restocked?

6. How can an assistant make an examination less stressful for a patient?

7. What principle must always be followed in assisting a patient to undress, as well as in draping for an examination?

B. Complete the following statements.
   1. The arranging of a sheet over a patient to prevent embarrassment but still allow the doctor to examine the patient is known as _____.

   2. When a patient's feet are placed into stirrups, this position is called the _____.

   3. The procedure carried out by the medical assistant before beginning any procedure on a patient and after the procedure is finished is _____.

   4. The position and the method of draping will depend upon _____ _____.

C. Fill in the blanks in column I with the correct answers from column II.

COLUMN I		COLUMN II	
1. _____	The patient lies flat on the abdomen with head turned right or left.	a.	horizontal recumbent
		b.	prone
2. _____	Position used for proctological examinations.	c.	Sims'
		d.	supine
3. _____	Also called stirrup position.	e.	dorsal recumbent
		f.	jackknife
4. _____	Patient lies flat on back with arms at side or across the chest.	g.	lateral
		h.	sitting
5. _____	The right arm and leg are flexed and the left arm and shoulder are front down on the table. The left leg is extended.		
6. _____	The patient is positioned at the side or end of the table with back straight and feet resting on stool.		

Unit 6 Examination Techniques

OBJECTIVES

After studying this unit, the student should be able to

- Describe the common methods of examination used during a physical examination.
- Name some routine laboratory tests which the doctor may order as part of the examination.
- Assemble the equipment necessary for a physical examination, a pelvic examination, and a rectal examination.

The assistant must be thoroughly familiar with the most common examination techniques in order to effectively assist the physician with examination and diagnostic procedures. This unit will introduce these techniques.

Many procedures are used to help the doctor determine what has caused the patient to become ill. By using the patient's history, physical examination, observations, and some specialized diagnostic procedures, such as laboratory tests and X rays, the doctor arrives at a diagnosis. The assistant will be helping the doctor carry out these diagnostic procedures. Therefore, it is vital that the assistant understand the techniques involved and be able to anticipate the doctor's actions.

A physical diagnosis is made by the doctor based upon conclusions made about the patient's condition. The physical assessment is made in four ways: by visual observations; palpation; auscultation; and percussion.

The first method used is *visual observation.* The doctor observes the patient's physical condition to see if the patient looks ill and, if so, what visible signs of illness are present.

The second method used is *palpation* (pal-pay-shun). By manual touch and pressure, the doctor feels parts of the body to find out if they are normal or not; he checks the size, shape, and consistency of the organs. This technique is used to determine the condition of internal organs that cannot be seen by visual observation.

The third method is *auscultation* (oz-cul-tay-shun). This is done by listening to certain parts of the body such as the heart or lungs and, sometimes, the abdominal area for sounds that indicate how these organs are functioning. A malfunction or poorly functioning organ can sometimes be detected by the sounds it makes. The doctor can use this information to help make a diagnosis.

The fourth method is *percussion* (per-kus-shun). The physician taps the body in a certain way placing one hand as a cushion on top of the part of the body being tapped by the other hand. By tapping the body (for example, the abdomen), listening to and feeling the local response, the doctor can often detect areas that are not functioning normally.

In addition to the four methods already discussed, the doctor may use laboratory results from examination of body fluids such as urine, blood, spinal fluid, feces, saliva, etc. Often X rays are necessary to make a definite diagnosis. Sometimes, it becomes necessary to remove small bits of tissue from the body and submit them to the clinical laboratory for study. This procedure is known as a *biopsy.*

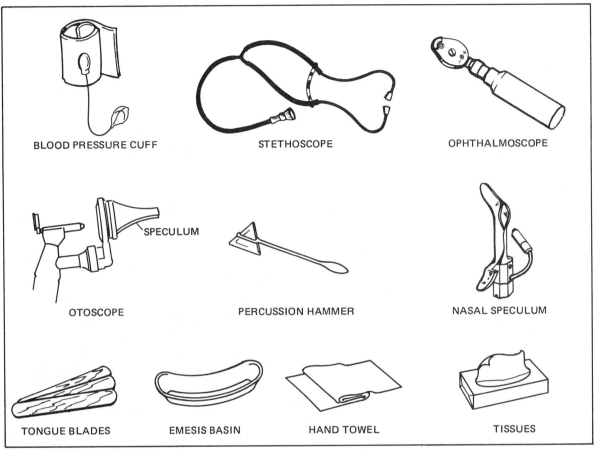

BLOOD PRESSURE CUFF

STETHOSCOPE

OPHTHALMOSCOPE

SPECULUM

OTOSCOPE

PERCUSSION HAMMER

NASAL SPECULUM

TONGUE BLADES

EMESIS BASIN

HAND TOWEL

TISSUES

Fig. 6-1 Items found on a physical exam tray.

Other diagnostic procedures which the doctor may use in special cases will be covered in the latter sections of the text.

The assistant's duties will vary in helping with diagnostic procedures. However, she must be familiar with the procedures and be able to prepare the patient and the examination room. The doctor will usually tell the medical assistant of any special equipment that might be needed in addition to the routine setup.

THE PHYSICAL EXAMINATION

After the physician has talked with the patient, he may tell the medical assistant to prepare to assist with the physical examination of the patient. Be sure the examining room has been cleaned and is ready to be set up and that the patient understands what is to be done.

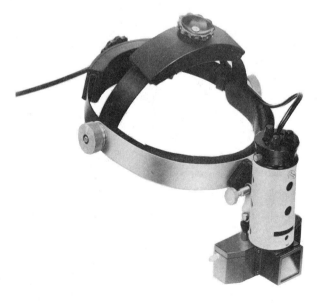

Fig. 6-2 Binocular indirect ophthalmoscope, used for close eye examinations.

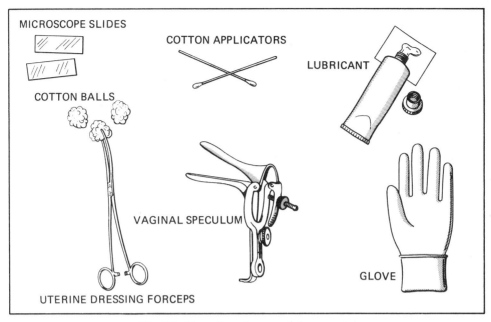

MICROSCOPE SLIDES

COTTON APPLICATORS

LUBRICANT

COTTON BALLS

VAGINAL SPECULUM

GLOVE

UTERINE DRESSING FORCEPS

Fig. 6-3 Items found on a pelvic exam tray.

A tray containing the following equipment will be needed for a physical examination, figure 6-1.

- Sphygmomanometer and stethoscope
- Ophthalmoscope (used to examine the eye)
- Otoscope (used to examine the ear)
- Percussion hammer (used to test reflexes)
- Nasal speculum
- Tongue blades
- Kidney or emesis basin
- Hand towel
- Tissues

Usually the patient will be placed in the supine or horizontal recumbent position and draped. The physician checks the abdomen and anterior (front) side of the body and then usually asks the patient to sit up for examination of the eyes, ears, nose, and throat. The doctor also checks the blood pressure, heart, lungs, and reflexes. When necessary, the assistant helps the patient into each position while avoiding unnecessary exposure of the patient's body. The assistant helps the doctor in any other way he requests keeping a close check on the equipment and supplies that need to be replaced.

If the physician wishes to perform a pelvic examination, the patient must be placed in the dorsal recumbent, or stirrup, position and draped. The equipment used for a pelvic examination, figure 6-3, will include the following.

- Disposable or rubber gloves
- Lubricant
- Vaginal speculum
- Long sponge forceps
- Cotton balls and applicators
- Slides, culture tubes, and other equipment used for doing a Papanicolaou (Pap's) smear.
- Good lighting (preferably a goose-neck lamp)
- Stool for the doctor

Be sure to test the light beforehand and replace bulb if necessary. Remember, the assistant remains in the room at all times when the doctor is examining a female patient. If an examination is taken of a child or a minor, the mother or another close relative should also be present.

All proctoscopic (prok-toe-skop-ik) examinations require cleansing of the rectum beforehand by means of enemas or laxatives. Instructions must be given to the patient who is scheduled for this examination. When a proctoscopic (rectal) examination is to be done, the assistant will place the patient in the jack-knife position, if the examining table will adjust to this position. If not, the knee-chest position is used; if the patient cannot maintain the knee-chest position because of age, weight, or some other reason, the lateral position may be used. The patient is properly draped and the physical setup prepared. The following equipment is used, figure 6-5. (As with all examinations, lighting must be pretested).

- Rectal speculum
- Disposable or rubber gloves
- Lubricant
- Cotton balls and applicators
- Proctoscope with light

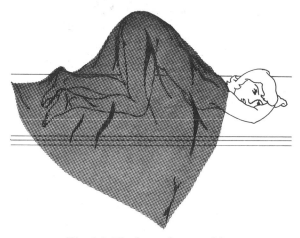

Fig. 6-4 The knee-chest position.

- Sigmoidoscope (if necessary)
- Stool for doctor

Remember, *always wash hands before beginning a procedure and immediately after the procedure.*

When the examination is finished, the assistant gently wipes off any lubricant that might have been used on the patient, helps the patient off the table, and helps her to dress, if needed. All equipment used must be thoroughly cleaned. The room must be clean and ready for the next patient.

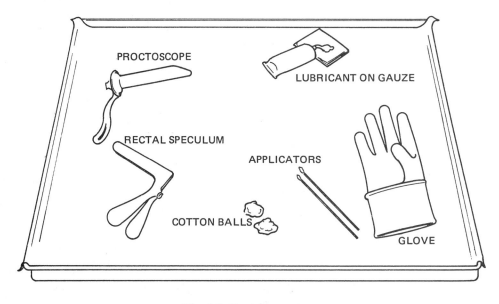

Fig. 6-5 Rectal exam tray.

SUMMARY

By knowing what techniques are used by the doctor, the assistant can set up the examining room and all equipment that will be needed. Each type of examination will require different types of setups. By thinking ahead, the assistant can prepare each patient and the physical setup without having to ask the doctor what is to be done. She should be able to anticipate what techniques will be used and what equipment will be needed. This makes assisting the doctor with the examinations much easier for all concerned; the patient, the doctor and the assistant.

Be sure the patient is aware of what is to be done, and that his questions have been answered. A cooperative patient makes physical examinations much easier.

Methods or techniques of physical examination are observation, palpation, auscultation, and percussion. Other examples of diagnostic techniques are laboratory examinations, x-ray examinations, and biopsies. The patient's medical history, the physical examination, and other diagnostic procedures are all used in helping the doctor to diagnose and treat the patient's illness or injury. The assistant must be familiar with all of the procedures and capable of assisting in the most efficient manner.

SUGGESTED ACTIVITIES

- Using outside references, write or give an oral report on the differences between the following types of diagnosis:

    Clinical diagnosis

    Physical diagnosis

    Differential diagnosis

- Using a medical dictionary, define the following words and study them so you can pronounce them correctly and understand their meanings.

    Prognosis

    Malignant

    Benign

    Terminal

    Therapy

    Pathology

REVIEW

Answer the following questions.

1. Name the term applied to procedures used by the physician to determine what is causing the patient to be ill.

2. Name the four methods used by the doctor to examine the patient during a physical examination.

3. Name five methods used by physicians to make a diagnosis.

4. Identify the procedure which involves removal of small bits of tissue from the body for laboratory studies.

5. List five body fluids that can be used to diagnose illness by laboratory methods.

6. List 8 pieces of equipment used for a physical examination setup.

7. List the equipment used for a pelvic tray setup.

8. How does the assistant's role differ when the patient for the physical examination is a minor or a child.

9. Name two positions which may be used for a rectal examination if the jackknife position cannot be used.

10. What equipment would be assembled for a rectal examination?

Self-Evaluation Test 1

Choose the answer that *best* completes the following statements.

1. The medical assistant is responsible to

    a. her doctor-employer for a well run, efficient office.
    b. her co-workers for harmony and co-operation.
    c. the patients for courteous, competent care.
    d. all of the above.

2. If injury to a patient resulted from the care given by a medical assistant, a lawsuit could be brought against

    a. the doctor.
    b. the medical assistant.
    c. all medical assistants employed in the office.
    d. the doctor and the medical assistant responsible.

3. The greatest fear is considered to be

    a. fear of dying.   c. fear of the unknown.
    b. fear of terminal illness.   d. all of these.

4. When the medical assistant establishes rapport with a patient, she

    a. is practicing medical ethics.
    b. eliminates all patient worry and anxiety.
    c. has built a link of communication and feeling with the patient.
    d. none of the above.

5. Body heat is produced in

    a. the alimentary canal.   c. the circulatory system.
    b. the body cells.   d. the bones.

6. The blood pressure, temperature, pulse, and respirations are called

    a. the vital signs.   c. both of these.
    b. signs of life.   d. neither of these.

7. The mouth, rectum and axilla are three sites used to measure

    a. blood pressure   c. pulse
    b. respiration   d. temperature

8. The pulse is usually taken at the

    a. brachial artery.   c. radial artery.
    b. brachial vein.   d. radial vein.

9. The systolic blood pressure is associated with

    a. cardiac contraction.   c. the cardiac cycle.
    b. cardiac relaxation.   d. all of these.

10. The sphygmomanometer is the apparatus used to

    a. measure the blood pressure.   c. count the pulse.
    b. listen to the blood pressure.   d. weigh the patient.

11. An abnormally slow pulse rate is called

    a. apnea.   c. cyanosis.
    b. bradycardia.   d. tachycardia.

12. High blood pressure is called

    a. tachycardia.   c. hypertension.
    b. bradycardia.   d. hypotension.

13. The lateral position used in examinations is also called the

    a. Sims' position.   c. Supine position.
    b. Jackknife position.   d. Prone position.

14. The following position is most often used for a proctological examination.

    a. Sitting position.   c. Dorsal recumbent position.
    b. Lateral position.   d. Jackknife position.

15. The special piece of equipment that is used to examine the ears is

    a. the ophthalmoscope.   c. the stethoscope.
    b. the otoscope.   d. the percussion hammer.

16. The procedures used by the physician to determine what is responsible for a patient's illness are called

    a. diagnostic procedures.   c. palpation.
    b. therapeutic procedures.   d. all of these.

17. Visible signs of illness are noted upon physical examination based on

    a. palpation.   c. clinical tests.
    b. observation.   d. auscultation.

18. Which of the following are not methods of diagnostic procedures?

    a. percussion and palpation.   c. X-ray and laboratory testing.
    b. auscultation and observation. d. therapeutic procedures.

19. A biopsy is

    a. a diagnostic procedure.
    b. a small bit of tissue removed from the body for clinical study.
    c. a method of examination.
    d. all of the above.

20. If a proctoscopic examination is to be done and the table will not adjust to a jackknife position, the position that may be used is the

    a. lateral position.   c. knee-chest position.
    b. supine position.   d. all but b.

Section 2
Aseptic Techniques

Unit 7 Microbiology

OBJECTIVES

After studying this unit, the student should be able to

- Identify three general groupings of bacteria according to their shapes.
- Define spores and explain their importance to the control and destruction of bacteria.
- Explain the relationship between bacteria and infection.

Microorganisms, or microbes, are tiny, primitive forms of life. Some microorganisms are necessary to life and some are harmful. This unit will identify some forms of microorganisms, how they cause infection, and how they are destroyed.

MICROORGANISMS

Most microorganisms are either tiny one-celled plants or animals. They can only be seen with a microscope. Algae, bacteria, and fungi are one-celled plants. They manufacture their food from their environment. One-celled animals cannot do this. They must obtain their food from other living things. The one-celled protozoa is an example of a one-celled animal.

A third group of microorganisms are viruses and rickettsiae. They have not been classified as either plant or animal due to their size which is too small even to be seen with any type of ordinary microscope. Research is underway to gain more information about these very small organisms.

Bacteria, which we are mainly concerned with, are usually classified according to the shape and arrangement of their cells when viewed through a microscope. There are three general groupings:

- Bacilli (rod-shaped)

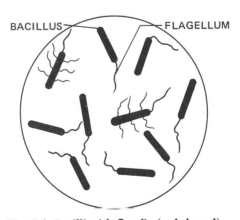

BACILLUS FLAGELLUM

Fig. 7-1 Bacilli with flagella (rod-shaped).

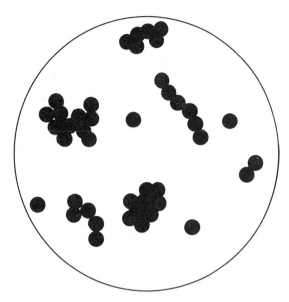

Fig. 7-2 Cocci (sphere-shaped).

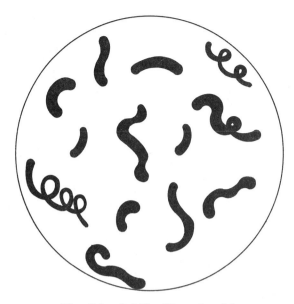

Fig. 7-3   Spirilla (Curved rods).

- Cocci (sphere-shaped)
- Spirilla (curved-rod)

The *bacilli* are rod-shaped cells which are straight and slender. Some are shaped like sausage or have tapering ends. Some bacilli have hairlike projections called flagella. These tails enable them to propel themselves about and achieve a small amount of movement.

Cocci are sphere-shaped cells that look like periods. If they are seen in pairs, they are *diplococci.* If they are viewed in a chain or string formation, they are *streptococci.* If they are arranged in clusters, they are *staphylococci,* figure 7-2.

The third group are called curved rods (or the *spirilla* group). These cells look like commas or corkscrews, figure 7-3. The comma-shaped rods are called *vibrio;* the corkscrew-shaped rods are called *spirilla.* Bacteria that are able to twist or move about are known as *spirochetes.*

Some bacteria can produce a starchy layer around the cell which helps to protect it. This is called a capsule. Bacteria that can form a covering around it that is tough enough to prevent anything from entering or leaving the cell

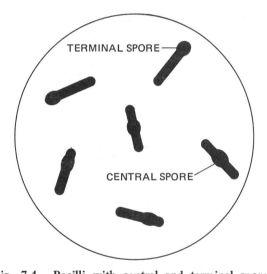

Fig. 7-4   Bacilli with central and terminal spores.

are called spore-forming bacteria. These bacteria are very difficult to kill because of this tough, protective covering. By forming spores, bacteria can become inactive until conditions are favorable for growth again. All of the spiral-shaped bacteria form spores and some of the rod-shaped bacteria can form spores. The spherical-shaped bacteria cannot form spores.

Bacteria are also either *aerobic* or *anaerobic* organisms. *Aerobic* bacteria must have free oxygen in order to survive, while *anaerobic* bacteria can only live where there is no oxygen.

Bacteria vary in the requirements necessary for life. These variables depend upon the type of bacteria under study. As already mentioned, some bacteria require oxygen, others do not; some grow best at high temperatures and others thrive on lower temperatures; some will need a slightly acid setting while others will need a slightly alkaline setting. Most bacteria require darkness to grow well; direct sunlight will kill some bacteria.

Bacteria is encouraged to grow in laboratory settings to be used for study and research. Optimal growing conditions are maintained in the laboratory. However, it is useful to know how to inhibit the growth of bacteria outside the laboratory. A dry atmosphere, excessive heat or cold, direct sunlight or ultraviolet light, and an extremely acid or alkaline environment will inhibit growth.

INFECTION

Infection occurs when disease-producing organisms enter the body and cause illness,

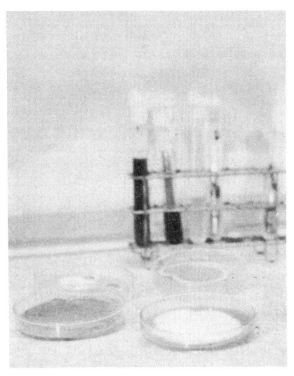

Fig. 7-5 Petri dishes and test tube cultures.

see Table 1. These microorganisms are called *pathogens.* They may enter the body through several routes. Airborne microbes may enter by way of the respiratory tract, or germs may be ingested or taken in through the digestive

CLASSIFICATION OF BACTERIA	SPECIFIC TYPE BACTERIA	DISEASE PRODUCED
BACILLI	tubercle bacillus	Tuberculosis
	bordetella pertussis	Pertussis (Whooping Cough)
	clostridium tetani	Tetanus
COCCI	gonococcus	Gonorrhea
	meningococcus	Meningitis (epidemic)
	pneumococcus	Pneumonia
	staphylococci	Impetigo and others
	streptococci	Scarlet fever, septicemia, and others
SPIRILLA	treponema pallidum	Syphilis
	borrelia Vincentii	Vincent's angina (trench mouth)
	vibrio comma	Cholera

Table 1 Pathogenic Bacteria.

tract. They may also enter through the urinary or reproductive systems, and through lacerations (cuts) or breaks in the skin.

When pathogens enter the body, disease may result. This is known as infection. If the infection remains in one area, it is a local infection. If it spreads to all parts of the body it is a systemic infection. Systemic or generalized infections are spread by the circulatory system.

Not all bacteria that enter the body cause infections. Many microbes are harmless and cause no damage to the person. Even pathogens do not always result in infections. If the body is normal and in good health, the body defenses will frequently kill the germs or render them harmless.

DESTRUCTION OF MICROBES

Microorganisms are everywhere. They thrive on the body surface and live in all the openings of the body. The mucous membranes lining the mouth and respiratory tract, as well as the digestive tract and the rectum and vagina harbor microorganisms. As long as the body's natural defenses are high, both pathogenic and nonpathogenic microbes can live there without causing infection. However, a lowered resistance caused by poor diet, fatigue or lack of fresh air and exercise will often result in infections. Only interior body tissues, that is, those that have no connection with the outside of the body, do not contain any bacteria (an example is the kidney).

The normal state of the atmosphere around us is such that microbes are almost always present. They are carried through the air on particles of dirt, dust, and moisture. They are also transferred by insects such as mosquitoes, flies, fleas, and lice, as well as rats, mice, and other animals. Person-to-person or direct contact also spreads microbes.

Due to the obvious abundance of microbes, some methods of controlling the growth and spread of these microbes are necessary. Aseptic techniques are methods that are used to kill and inhibit the growth of these microorganisms. It is absolutely necessary for the medical assistant to learn these methods and to be skilled in their use in order to prevent contamination and the spread of infection and disease. Care must be taken in using these techniques so that the patients as well as the assistant and the other office personnel are protected.

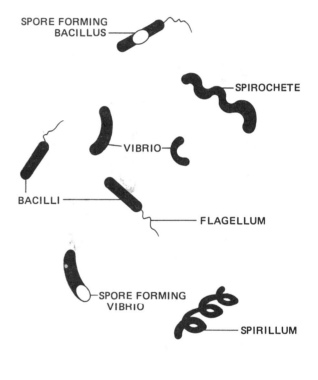

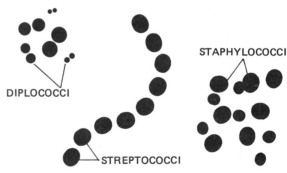

Fig. 7-6 Various forms of bacteria.

Antisepsis is the prevention of any further growth of microbes. *Antiseptics* do not kill bacteria or germs; they simply inhibit their growth and cause the microbes to be in a state of *bacteriostasis* which means they cannot multiply or reproduce. The medication placed on wounds or cuts are usually antiseptics.

Disinfection is a process that kills all pathogenic organisms except the spore-forming bacteria. A *bactericide* or *germicide* is a chemical agent which will kill bacteria that are pathogenic. Iodine and carbolic acid (phenol) are frequently used as disinfectants.

Sterilization is a method of killing every living microorganism. This process is used in hospitals, doctor's offices, or any situation where absolute absence of microbes is necessary to avoid infection. Sterilization is achieved by using extremely high dry heat or live steam under pressure. Boiling will kill some pathogens but, since spore-forming pathogens are very difficult to destroy, it is best to use steam under pressure to ensure destruction of all pathogens.

SUMMARY

Microorganisms come in various shapes and all arrangements, figure 7-6; they are tiny one-celled plants or animals which may cause disease. They can enter the body by way of the respiratory, digestive, urinary, reproductive tracts, or through breaks in the skin; this can result in infection.

Methods of controlling microbial growth are sterilization, disinfection, and antisepsis. Autoclaving (steam heat under pressure) is the surest method of destroying the living microorganisms.

SUGGESTED ACTIVITIES

- Using five sterile petri dishes containing agar which have been prepared by the instructor, try the following experiments:

    1. One student touches a sterile petri dish with her finger.
    2. Another student touches a dish with her nose.
    3. Another student touches a dish with the tip of her tongue.
    4. A student breathes on a dish.
    5. A student coughs on a dish.

    All plates should be labeled and incubated until growth can be seen. A slide is then made of the material from each plate by the instructor. The students view the microbial growth through a microscope.

- Mix some common household antiseptics and disinfectants with the agar and label the dishes before sterilization. Compare the growth on the plates containing the antiseptics and disinfectants with the previously prepared plates. Observe how the antiseptics and disinfectants affect the microbial growth.

REVIEW

A. Completion items

   1. Microorganisms are either one-celled _____ or _____ with the exception of the _____ and _____.

2. Bacteria are usually classified according to _____ and _____.

3. Describe the shape of the following bacteria.

   a. bacilli _____

   b. cocci _____

   c. vibrio _____

   d. spirilla _____

B. Answer the following questions.

1. Define the following terms.

   a. capsule

   b. spore

2. List the spore-producing bacteria.

3. What is the difference in aerobic and anaerobic bacteria?

4. List four variables related to bacterial growth.

5. What does the term "optimal growth conditions" mean?

6. What is the difference between a pathogenic organism and a non-pathogenic organism?

7. What determines whether a microbe will cause an infection or not?

8. Name five ways bacteria can enter the body.

9. Infections affect the body in two ways. Name them.

10. What part of the body has no microorganisms?

11. Name some ways microbes are carried from one place to another.

12. List and briefly define the three methods of controlling the growth and spread of microbes.

C. 1. Label the bacteria on diagram A.

DIAGRAM A

2. Identify the specific cocci shown in diagram B.

DIAGRAM B

Unit 8 Microbial Control

OBJECTIVES

After studying this unit, the student should be able to

- Explain why microbial control is necessary and why the assistant must practice it.
- Define asepsis and sepsis; medical and surgical asepsis.
- List the four methods of sterilization.
- State the differences between sanitization, disinfection, and sterilization.

The medical assistant must learn what microbial control is and how it is achieved. There are several methods as discussed briefly in the previous unit. All medical personnel must have a thorough understanding of how microorganisms are spread and how they are controlled and destroyed.

PURPOSE

Microbial control is necessary to prevent the spread of illness and infectious or contagious diseases. The medical assistant will come into contact with many different kinds of diseases, illnesses, and injuries. Many of these conditions will be caused and transmitted by microorganisms. Therefore, the medical assistant must learn how to control and destroy these pathogenic organisms.

Diseases that are spread by microorganisms are said to be contagious or communicable diseases. The doctor's office can become a meeting place and breeding ground for germs unless proper precautions are observed by everyone at all times. The importance of conscientious practice of good techniques cannot be stressed enough.

Proper techniques of medical and surgical asepsis are routine but very necessary procedures in the office. *Asepsis* means without dirt or germs. *Septic* means dirty and con-

taminated. *Medical asepsis* includes sanitization and disinfection procedures that are vital to patient protection. Surgical asepsis is also a part of patient protection but is more thorough and results in sterile (without any living organism) procedures performed instead of simply clean, safe procedures.

SANITIZATION

Sanitization is thorough cleansing of all facilities, homes, public places, and other areas used by people. Sanitization is the method of cleanliness practiced in homes and by all people concerned with prevention and spread or microorganisms. This includes sanitation departments, garbage disposal agencies, public health departments, city and county health departments, the medical team, and all citizens. Remember, bacteria thrive in warm, dark, damp places. Any area that might result in disease producing organisms that could cause poor health is a concern to all.

One of the primary aids to cleanliness and sanitation is handwashing. While soap and water handwashing will not kill germs or even inhibit their growth as antiseptics and disinfectants do, it does remove many of the germs. Soap reduces the surface tension of the skin; the running water washes away the dirt and germs that are loosened by the friction

CHEMICAL AGENT	STRENGTH	USAGE
Phenol	0.5 to 1%	Antiseptic strength but may be irritating and toxic to tissue.
	5% (standard)	Disinfection of utensils, facilities, and human excreta.
	88%	To cauterize small wounds.
Lysol	1 to 2%	Antiseptic cleanser for hands.
	2 to 5%	Disinfectant: facilities and contaminated items.
Mercury Bichloride	1:2,000 to 1:20,000	Disinfect hands or wounds (Poisonous)
Mercurochrome	1%	Urinary antiseptic (aqueous solution)
	2%	Skin antiseptic
Merthiolate	1:1,000	Skin disinfection (tincture)
	1:1,000	Disinfectant for instruments (Aq. Sol.)
Zephiran Chloride	1:1,000	Disinfectant for rubber and metal instruments.
	1:2,000 to	Skin and wound disinfectant and antiseptic.
	1:10,000	(Dependent upon strength.)
Alcohol	70%	Skin and instrument disinfectant.

Fig. 8-1 Some common chemical agents.

that is created when the hands are rubbed together. Soap does not kill germs. In doctor's offices, dry soap or soap dispensers of some kind are used.

Hands should be washed thoroughly from the wrists down, using a soft brush and soap dispensed from a container. Warm running water is necessary to wash the dirt and germs away. Paper towels are best for drying since they can be used once and thrown away. Damp linen towels can transmit microbes. Hands should be washed before beginning any procedure on a patient and after each patient has been cared for. This serves to protect the patients from transmission of microbes by direct contact and protects the assistant as well. The assistant should never touch the area in or around her mouth or face. This is a good policy to follow at all times.

DESTRUCTION OF ORGANISMS

Disinfection is a process that will usually kill all pathogenic organisms except spore-forming ones. There are many germicidal or bactericidal chemical agents available to health workers. Although these agents will kill pathogenic microbes they do not necessarily destroy nonpathogenic organisms. Many of the chemical agents used are diluted with another liquid to make them safe to use.

Antiseptic solutions are weak and may be used safely on the skin and, in some cases, inside the body. Disinfecting solutions are much stronger and are never used inside the body because of danger of chemical burns and tissue damage. Disinfectants are used for killing pathogenic bacteria (with the exception of spores) on instruments and equipment. Disinfectants are also used for cleaning areas in the office. The strength used for sterilizing instruments by soaking them for a given period of time would be much greater than the strength used on floors, cabinets, bathrooms, etc. The antiseptic strengths are not strong enough to kill bacteria. However, they do inhibit the growth and reproduction of microbes. This classifies them as *bacteriostatic* solutions rather than germicidal solutions as are the disinfectants.

TYPE OF STERILIZATION	METHOD USED	TIME REQUIRED	EFFECTIVENESS
Chemical	Strong disinfectant solution	20 to 30 minutes	Fair. Kills most microorganisms except spores.
Dry Heat 150°C	Hot air oven	One hour minimum	Poor. Uncertain and doesn't kill spores.
Boiling 100°C	Office sterilizer	20 to 30 minutes	Good. Kills all microorganisms except spores.
Steam under pressure 15 lbs. @ 121.6°C	Autoclave	15 to 30 minutes	Excellent. Kills all microorganisms including spores.

Fig. 8-2 Sterilization guidelines.

Phenol (carbolic acid) is the chemical frequently used as a disinfectant in medical settings; it is used in varying strengths for different purposes. Even commercially prepared disinfectants must be handled carefully and used as directed since phenol solutions and other disinfectants may cause burns if handled improperly. Phenol forms the base for many solutions whether prepared commercially or mixed in the hospital or clinic. The U.S. Pure Food and Drug Administration has determined that phenol is to be used as a standard for testing the killing strength of disinfectants. This is known as the *phenol coefficient* and is used as standard for testing and classifying disinfectants.

STERILIZATION

This process kills all microbes including pathogens, nonpathogens, and spores. It can be achieved or carried out by several methods. Some methods are far safer and more reliable than others.

Cold temperatures are not a method of killing microorganisms. Freezing will retard the growth of some bacteria and prevent their reproduction and spread. Freezing is useful in food preservation as it prevents the bacteria from growing and causing the food to spoil, but it is of little or no use in sterilization.

Light can be used in some cases to kill bacteria. Sunlight will inhibit the growth of

bacteria; ultraviolet rays may kill bacteria if exposed long enough. Ultraviolet lighting is used in hospitals to destroy some airborne bacteria in some areas such as newborn nurseries and operating rooms.

Chemical sterilization can be achieved by soaking instruments and some other types of equipment in a very strong disinfectant solution for a given period of time. The time will depend upon the type of solution used. This method will kill pathogenic organisms but not spores.

Heat is the most effective method of sterilization. However, the use of heat alone is not always sufficient. Time and the type of heat used are important variables. Some microorganisms require much higher temperatures for a longer period of time to ensure their

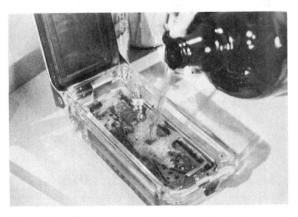

Fig. 8-3 Chemical sterilization; the instruments should be completely covered with the germicide in a glass container.

destruction than do others. The spores can withstand very high temperatures for long periods of time if the heat is dry heat. For example, to sterilize instruments using the dry heat method (hot air ovens) would require temperatures in excess of 150° Celsius or 302° Fahrenheit for a minimum of one hour to kill bacteria. This still would not kill the spores.

Moist heat is more effective in sterilization than dry heat. Boiling water is one simple, safe method of sterilization. However, it is more time consuming than live steam under pressure; also some articles cannot be boiled. If the articles are completely covered with boiling water at 100°C or 212°F and maintained at that temperature for a least 20 minutes, all bacteria except spores will be destroyed. To kill spores, the articles would have to be boiled for thirty minutes daily on three consecutive days.

The best and most efficient method of sterilization is live steam under pressure. The *autoclave* is the means by which this is accomplished. It works on the same principles as a pressure cooker. Because the steam is under pressure the temperatures reached are much higher than the temperature of boiling water. The time required to kill all bacteria, including spores, is less than that of boiling or chemical sterilization. At 15 pounds of pressure and 121.6°C all bacteria are killed within 15 to 30 minutes. This is the method of sterilization used in hospitals, clinics, and most doctor's offices. Autoclaves range is sizes from small tabletop units to large walk-in units used in hospitals.

SUMMARY

Sanitization and disinfection are both important parts of medical asepsis. Asepsis refers to procedures and methods used to ensure the prevention and spread of microbes. These measures are important for the protection of the patients and the staff. Microorganisms are spread by direct and indirect methods of transmission.

Surgical asepsis includes sterilization procedures which kill disease-producing organisms. There are several sterilization methods used such as chemical sterilization, dry heat, moist heat, and live steam under pressure. The autoclave which is the live steam under pressure method, is the safest and most efficient. It is the only method that ensures the destruction of all bacteria, including spores, within a reasonable amount of time.

SUGGESTED ACTIVITIES

- Make arrangements for a visit to a hospital's central supply department or the OR (operating room) for a demonstration of sterilization procedures.

- Arrange a visit to the local water control board for a demonstration of how water is kept sanitary and safe for drinking.

- Using outside resources, write a short report on pasteurization. Document the report with the sources of information.

- In small groups, discuss methods of sanitization and disinfection that are frequently used in the home. Include any instances where sterilization could be used.

REVIEW

A.   Briefly answer the following questions.

1. Why is microbial control necessary?

2. What is sanitization?

3. What is antisepsis?

4. What is a term used that describes the effect of antiseptic solutions.

5. What purpose does soap serve in handwashing?

6. What is disinfection?

7. List the four methods of sterilization.

8. What is the difference between sterilization and disinfection?

9. Which is the most effective method of sterilization? Why?

10. What is another name for Phenol?

11. What is a chemical solution?

12. What is meant by the phenol coefficient?

13. a. What effect does a freezing temperature have upon bacteria?

    b. When is this useful?

14. What effect does sunlight have on bacteria?

15. What effect does an ultraviolet light have on bacteria?

16. List two important ways that antiseptics and disinfectants differ.

17. What is contamination and how does it occur?

B. Complete the following.

1. To sterilize articles, the autoclave must heat to _____ degrees under _____ pounds of pressure for _____ minutes.

2. To kill bacteria except spores, a dry heat oven would have to maintain _____ degrees of heat for _____ minutes.

3. Boiling water must reach _____ degrees of heat for at least _____ minutes to kill bacteria except the _____ bacteria.

4. What would happen if someone dropped instruments into a boiling water sterilizer where you had already begun boiling instruments 10 minutes earlier? _____

5. Make a chart of the methods of sterilization, beginning with the least effective. List the time required to achieve sterilization.

Method	time required

6. What strength of carbolic acid is used as a standard disinfectant? _____

7. What strength of Lysol solution is used as an antiseptic for the hands? _____

Unit 9 The Autoclave

OBJECTIVES

After studying this unit, the student should be able to

- Describe how an autoclave operates, based on steam pressure and steam flow.
- Name and give the use of autoclave gauges.
- Prepare materials for autoclave sterilization.
- Demonstrate how to operate an autoclave.

The autoclave is the machine that is used for the sterilization method, using steam under pressure. It works on the same principles as a home pressure cooker. The medical assistant must know the principles of autoclave use, how to prepare packs for sterilization, and how to load the autoclave.

DESCRIPTION AND PRINCIPLES

The autoclave consists of an outer jacket surrounding a sterilizing chamber. A water source allows water to be turned into steam by the heating elements. When the proper amount of pressure has been achieved (usually 15 pounds of pressure per square inch) the jacket is opened automatically so that the steam flows into the upper rear of the chamber.

As the steam flows into the rear of the chamber, the air already inside is forced out through a valve in the lower, front area. A thermometer is located at the air outlet valve so that the reading given is always that of the lowest temperature in the sterilizing chamber. When all air has been evacuated, the temperature will begin to rise, and the air valve will automatically close.

There are several gauges located on an autoclave. One is the temperature gauge. This will indicate the lowest temperature in the chamber. Another gauge will give the pounds of pressure reading in pounds per square inch. Still other gauges will indicate how long the autoclave has been operating at a preset temperature and pressure and serves as a timer.

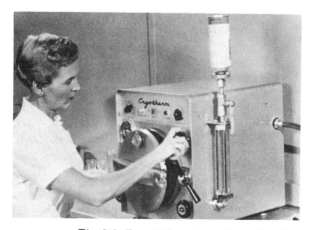 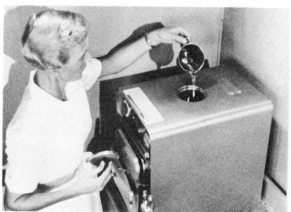

Fig. 9-1 Two different autoclaves based on same principles. (Courtesy Wyeth Laboratories)

There may be other dials and gauges on autoclaves depending on what kind and model is used.

NOTE: Timing for a sterilization procedure does not begin until both the pressure and temperature has reached the required minimums. Pressure must be 15 pounds per square inch and temperature must be 250° to 254° Fahrenheit.

After the sterilization is completed, the autoclave must be vented. This allows the pressure to drop and the chamber to cool; this is usually done automatically. The door has an automatic, safety lock which will prevent the opening of the door as long as there is pressure in the chamber. Steam under pressure can cause serious injuries; never try to force an autoclave door open. It should remain locked until the pressure has been vented and the chamber has had time to become dry and cool. *The complete directions for use of any autoclave should be read before operating it.*

ADVANTAGES

The advantages of autoclaving have been discussed in previous units but will be repeated because of the importance of asepsis.

One of the most obvious advantages of the autoclave's use is its effectiveness. All living organisms are killed after a 10 minute exposure to 250°F under 15 pounds of pressure. Even the most difficult to destroy (spores) are killed in 20 to 30 minutes.

Many different types of articles can be sterilized at the same time in an autoclave. Bottled liquids can be sterilized at the same time that instruments and supplies are being processed. If this is done, the instruments and supplies should be packaged.

Using sterile indicators, such as autoclave tape, will assure that the articles processed are actually sterile. This tape has very faint mark-

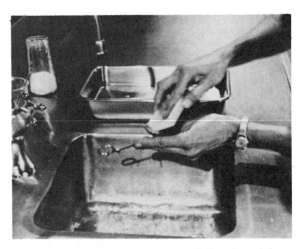

Fig. 9-2 Cleaning instruments with brush and low-sudsing detergent.

ings that become very pronounced when the sterilization process is complete. These markings may change colors or just become much darker. Directions will be included with any type of sterile indicators. This tape is also convenient for writing the date of sterilization for future use.

USING THE AUTOCLAVE

All articles to be autoclaved must first be thoroughly cleaned. Instruments are washed carefully with a low-sudsing detergent and a stiff brush, rinsed completely, and dried. Care must be taken while washing the instruments to remove all blood or other substances. Instruments that are hinged should be autoclaved in the open position. Instruments may be autoclaved on a tray if they are not to be used in sterile packs. Any article that must remain sterile after autoclaving should be wrapped in a special way to maintain sterility. This will be covered later.

Jars, cans, or containers must be placed on their sides, uncovered, so that the steam can penetrate to the insides of the containers and the covers. Remember, the cool, dry air is forced downward and out through the exhaust valve; the steam is moving from above in a downward movement of flow.

Packs are placed on their sides to allow steam to freely penetrate the area between trays and articles. If liquids are being sterilized, the containers should not be tightly capped but closed with a large roll of gauze pads, figure 9-3. The cover should also be autoclaved. After the articles are removed from the autoclave, the gauze pads are carefully removed and the sterile cover put in place. Sterile technique must be used in this procedure.

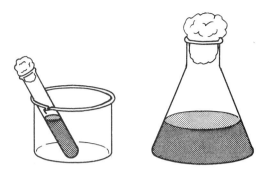

Fig. 9-3 Solutions ready for sterilization.

PACKS

Articles that need to remain sterile after autoclaving must be wrapped properly and taped with an autoclave indicator tape. Either a cloth material or 2-3 layers of disposable paper may be used to wrap packs. If cloth is used, it should be clean and unwrinkled. Today most packs are wrapped in disposable paper wraps. The wrap must allow steam to penetrate to the inside in order to sterilize the articles.

Wrappings are to serve as barriers for contaminants during storage and handling. Wrappings must remain dry at all times after sterilization. A sterile pack that becomes damp or wet after sterilization also becomes contaminated. This is one reason why packs are not removed from the autoclave until they are cool and dry.

Articles may be wrapped singly or in groups that will be used together at the same time, for example, dressing trays or suture packs. (A *suture pack* includes all the necessary articles needed to suture or stitch a cut or laceration except the silk or catgut used to close the wound.)

When wrapping an article or a pack for the autoclave, the wrap is placed flat on a smooth surface. Clean, dry articles are placed in the center and the bottom edge of the wrap is folded up over the articles, figure 9-4. The corner of the wrap is turned down and folded. The left side is then folded over to the right and the tip of the corner is folded back to the left. The right side

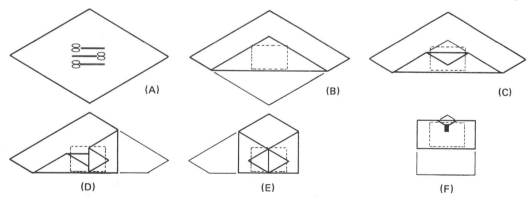

Fig. 9-4 Wrapping articles for the autoclave: (A) Place all items in center and (B) fold linen up from bottom, (C) doubling back a small corner. (D) Fold over the right, (E) and then the left, edges. Leave the corners doubled back. (F) Fold the pack up from the bottom and secure it with pressure-sensitive tape. (Courtesy of Wyeth Laboratories)

Table A Sterilization Time For The Autoclave	
ARTICLE	**TIME**
Glass syringes	30 minutes
Instruments, unwrapped	15 minutes
Instruments, surgical, opened	15 minutes
Instruments, wrapped in packs	30 minutes
Surgical scrub brushes	15 minutes
Rubber gloves	15 minutes
Solutions in flasks with gauze stopper	30 minutes
Glassware	30 minutes
Enamel or stainless steel articles	20 minutes
Hypodermic needles, wrapped	20 minutes
Small packs, wrapped	20 minutes
Large packs, wrapped	20 minutes

is folded toward the left with the tip folded back to the right. The top edge is folded down with the tip folded up. The tips are folded in the opposite direction from the fold so that the packs may be opened without contaminating the interior of the sterile packs. When the last fold has been completed, the wrap is secured with autoclave tape and dated. The date is important as articles will not remain sterile indefinitely even though they are properly wrapped. The tape should always be checked when packs are removed from the autoclave to be sure sterilization has taken place. When stored, the packs should be checked periodically and re-autoclaved if necessary.

Even when using the autoclave, time is a factor which may vary according to the type of material and articles being sterilized. The table of sterilization time required for some articles should be studied for comparisons.

SUMMARY

The autoclave works on the same principle as the pressure cooker. Water is turned into steam under pressure and the combination of high temperatures and pressure kill all living organisms including spores. Timing of sterilization does not begin until the temperature and pressure have reached required levels.

In order for complete sterilization to be achieved, packs must be properly wrapped and placed in the autoclave. Autoclave tape is used to ensure that sterilization has occured. Packs and all other articles must be placed in the autoclave in a manner that will allow the steam to circulate freely and reach all surfaces of all articles.

Articles are never removed from the autoclave until they have been cooled and dried. This usually occurs automatically. The door remains locked until the process is complete. Never try to force an autoclave door open. Live steam can cause severe burns.

SUGGESTED ACTIVITIES

- Make a diagrammatic chart of the flow of air and steam in the autoclave.

- Practice wrapping various size packs for the autoclave. Have the instructor check each pack.

- Using outside resources, write a short report on how pressure affects temperature.

REVIEW

Briefly answer the following questions.

1. The autoclave works on the same principle as what common, home utensil?

2. What single factor makes the autoclave more effective than any other type of sterilization?

3. What does the thermometer reading at the air outlet valve represent?

4. Describe the directional flow of steam as it enters the autoclave chamber.

5. Describe the directional flow of air as it enters the autoclave chamber.

6. List three kinds of gauges that might be found on an autoclave.

7. What procedure must be carried out on all articles before they are wrapped and placed into the autoclave?

8. List three advantages of using an autoclave.

9. What is meant by the term, *venting?*

10. How should hinged instruments be positioned in the autoclave?

11. What is a pack?

12. Why are articles placed in a wrapper before autoclaving?

13. How should jars, cans, or containers be positioned in the autoclave to ensure sterilization? Why?

14. What are the two kinds of wrappers that are used to prepare packs for sterilization in the autoclave?

15. List three ways that sterile articles may become contaminated.

Unit 10 The Sterilizer

OBJECTIVES

After studying this unit, the student should be able to

- List the advantages and disadvantages of a sterilizer.
- Give the time and temperature necessary to kill pathogenic organisms (other than spores) in sterilizer.
- Explain why the destruction of spores is not practical in a sterilizer.
- Sterilize various types of articles using an office sterilizer.

The physician's office usually has a small sterilizer, in addition to the autoclave. These sterilizers are filled with water that is boiled by an electrical unit. They are used to sterilize small articles that will not be harmed by boiling procedures. The medical assistant must learn to use and care for the office sterilizer.

DESCRIPTION AND PRINCIPLES

Boiling some articles will kill living organisms that are present on them. One method of boiling is the use of the small office sterilizer, a stainless steel machine that contains water and an electrical unit that heats the water to boiling temperature. It also has a hinged lid that is attached to a tray. The tray is lowered into the boiling water when the lid of the sterilizer is closed. Some of the older types of sterilizers have trays that must be lifted out by hand; these must be handled with great care to prevent burning the hands.

The water is heated to a temperature of 100°Celsius (212°Fahrenheit) and maintained at that temperature for the length of time required to sterilize the articles inside the sterilizer. The time will vary according to the articles placed in the unit.

ADVANTAGES

One of the foremost advantages of the sterilizer is that it is quick and easy to use. No wrapping or preparation of packs is necessary.

Another advantage is that it is more economical and faster than using the autoclave if

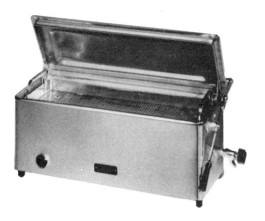

Fig. 10-1 The office sterilizer.

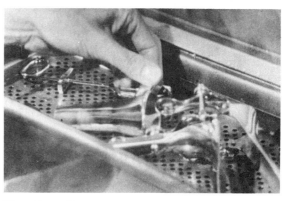

Fig. 10-2 Placing clean instruments in a sterilizer.
(Courtesy Wyeth labs)

there are only one or two articles to be sterilized.

USE OF THE STERILIZER

The office sterilizer is most frequently used for sterilizing small, blunt instruments (boiling dulls sharp instruments), soft-rubber goods, and small pieces of glassware.

The articles to be sterilized must first be cleaned with soap and water and thoroughly rinsed. Any blood that remains should be removed with a brush and special solvent. Be sure that all soap is rinsed off articles before placing them in the sterilizer. It is not necessary that they be dry. All articles to be sterilized are placed on the tray and lowered into the boiling water.

The sterilizer will have some means of indicating when the water has again reached the boiling temperature after the articles have been placed inside. A red light is most frequently used to indicate that the water is at boiling temperature. NOTE: Timing does not begin until this indicator shows that boiling temperature has been reached. After timing has begun, nothing else should be added to the sterilizer until the cycle is completed. If something must be added, the timing cycle must begin again when the temperature has reached boiling after the addition of the last articles.

If the instruments are to be used while still sterile, they must be carefully removed from the sterilizer with sterile transfer forceps using sterile technique. Great care must be taken to see that the instruments remain sterile and do not become contaminated during the transfer. Remember, these articles will be very hot when they are lifted out of the sterilizer.

If it is not necessary that the instruments remain sterile, they can be allowed to cool either in the tray or while resting on a clean, dry surface such as a clean hand towel. Many

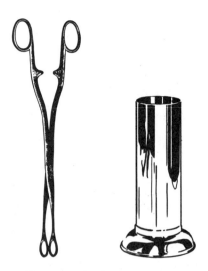

Fig. 10-3 Transfer forceps and container.

times, the sterilizer will be used to kill pathogenic organisms that might have contaminated the articles during patient use. These articles do not necessarily have to be sterile for patient use but should be clean and free from pathogenic organisms. An example of this situation might be forceps used while changing a dressing on a patient but not actually used in contact with the patient's skin or tissue. Another example would be the speculums used in examining the nose. These instruments are sterilized after each use. Since the inside of the nose is not a sterile area, the speculum must be clean and free from all pathogenic germs, however, the speculum may be stored in a clean, dry, dust-free area. They will remain clean but not sterile when stored this way for future use.

The following chart gives the sterilization time for different types of articles.

Soft rubber goods (never boiled with other articles)	15 minutes
Small blunt metal instruments (opened if hinged)	20 minutes
Small glass articles (syringes, medicine glasses)	20 minutes

Since tap water usually leaves a residue or sediment when boiled, the sterilizer must be cleaned frequently. This is necessary at least once a week and sometimes more often. To clean the sterilizer, one cup of household vinegar or other cleaner specified by the manufacturer is added to the water. Boil for at least 30 minutes. Pour out the solution and remove any residue that might remain by gently scraping the inside of the sterilizer. Wipe down the inside of the sterilizer with 70% alcohol.

Remember, the sterilizer will kill living organisms except for spore-forming bacteria. Spore-forming bacteria will survive boiling and should be autoclaved in order to ensure their destruction.

SUMMARY

The sterilizer is used in the doctor's office to kill most microorganisms. Articles which will come into direct contact with the patient's tissue should be autoclaved because spore-forming bacteria cannot be destroyed by the sterilizer method.

Articles that have become contaminated by microorganisms (other than the spore-forming ones) should be washed and rinsed, then sterilized by boiling to kill the living organisms that might be transmitted to another patient. If an article is to be used immediately and should be sterile, it is transferred to a sterile setting using special techniques to prevent contamination. Articles sterilized in a small sterilizer are stored in a clean, dust-free place.

SUGGESTED ACTIVITIES

- In discussion groups, review the following articles and decide whether or not they would be sterilized in a boiling water sterilizer. If not, would they be autoclaved?

rubber gloves	disposable needles
plastic tubing	razor blades or knife blades
suture scissors	percussion hammer

REVIEW

Briefly answer the following questions.

1. What temperature must be maintained through the sterilization procedure when the boiling method is used?

2. Using a small office sterilizer, how would you know when the proper temperature had been reached?

3. When does timing begin when using the sterilizer or boiling method?

4. List two advantages of using the sterilizer.

5. What three kinds of instruments or articles are most often sterilized by the boiling method? List the time required for each.

6. What types of instruments are not placed in the office sterilizer or in any boiling water? Why?

7. What must be done to any article before placing it into the sterilizer?

8. Why is it necessary to sterilize articles that do not have to be sterile to be used?

9. Would this type of sterilization procedure be called medical or surgical asepsis?

10. What is the purpose of this asepsis?

11. Where would articles be stored if they do not have to be kept sterile?

12. What microorganisms are not destroyed by boiling in an office sterilizer?

Unit 11 Chemical Sterilization

OBJECTIVES

After studying this unit, the student should be able to

- List the advantages and disadvantages of chemical sterilization.
- Relate the effectiveness of chemical sterilization against spores.
- List some chemicals used in chemical sterilization and their advantages and disadvantages.

Chemical sterilization, or cold sterilization as it is often referred to, is the immersion of instruments and small articles in a chemical solution of high germicidal action. The medical assistant must learn to disinfect and to sterilize by this method.

DESCRIPTION AND PRINCIPLES

The use of disinfectant solutions has already been discussed and must be understood in order to effectively deal with chemical or cold sterilization. Disinfecting solutions are strong, chemical solutions that kill pathogenic organisms.

Disinfectant solutions are limited in their use since they do not destroy nonpathogens or spores. The assistant should be aware of these limitations when using the chemical sterilization method. Usually, the assistant must rely upon the claims of commercial manufacturers which, in turn, are subject to regulations.

Chemical sterilization is most often used for convenience. It is the preferred means of killing pathogens on articles that may be damaged by heat.

USE OF CHEMICAL STERILIZATION

A good chemical solution for disinfection or sterilization should be effective in weak concentrations. It should remain effective while it is working and not lose its potency

because of exposure to certain kinds of materials. It should not be damaging to tissues. Many effective disinfecting solutions are very *caustic;* that is, they are damaging to tissues.

The chemical solution used should be placed in an airtight container. The directions for the use of that particular chemical should be followed carefully. Instruments or small articles that are to be sterilized in this manner are thoroughly cleaned. In addition to careful cleaning with soap and water, they must be rinsed completely free of any type of soap or cleaning solution. They must be dried thoroughly in order to avoid diluting the chemical solution and decreasing its effectiveness.

After this cleaning procedure, the articles are carefully placed in the chemical solution in a container with an airtight cover; they are left

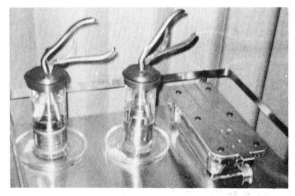

Fig. 11-1 Chemical sterilization: Two sterile forceps in airtight jars; sterile tray containing a chemical solution.

CHEMICAL AGENT	STRENGTH	USAGE
Phenol	0.5 to 1% 5% (standard) 88%	Antiseptic strength but may be irritating and toxic to tissue. Disinfection of utensils, facilities, and human excreta. To cauterize small wounds.
Lysol	1 to 2% 2 to 5%	Antiseptic cleanser for hands. Disinfectant: facilities and contaminated items.
Mercury Bichloride	1 : 2,000 to 1 : 20,000	Disinfect hands or wounds (POISONOUS)
Mercurochrome	1% 2%	Urinary antiseptic. (Aqueous solution) Skin antiseptic.
Merthiolate	1 : 1,000 1 : 1,000	Skin disinfection. (Tincture) Disinfectant for instruments. (Aq. Sol.)
Zephiran Chloride	1 : 1,000 1 : 2,000 to 1 : 10,000	Disinfectant for rubber and metal instruments. Skin and wound disinfectant and antiseptic. (Dependent upon strength.)
Alcohol	70%	Skin and instrument disinfectant.

Fig. 11-2 Some common chemical agents.

in this solution, undisturbed, for 20 to 30 minutes in most cases. Again, the assistant is reminded to read the instructions on commercially prepared solutions for time requirements.

The solution used for sterilization purposes should remain uncontaminated. This means that sterile pick-up forceps must be used to remove articles after their allotted time in the solution. The same principles apply to chemical sterilization (sometimes called cold sterilization) that apply to sterilization by boiling. If the instruments are being sterilized mainly to kill pathogenic organisms and are not to be used in sterile procedures, they can be dried and stored in a clean, dry, dust-free area. If the instruments are to be used in a sterile procedure, they must be removed with pick-up forceps, placed on a sterile tray and used immediately.

COMMONLY USED CHEMICALS

Alcohol 70% solution is the most widely used disinfectant. As its concentration increases, the effectiveness decreases so that 99% alcohol is ineffective as a disinfectant agent; 70% isopropl alcohol is effective and noncaustic or damaging to tissues. However, alcohol will cause rusting of delicate instruments and some other metallic articles.

Phenol is frequently used in weak dilutions but it remains very caustic and is most often mixed with some other chemical agent.

Formaldehyde or formalin is a very strong disinfectant and is also used as a tissue preservative. If it is mixed in the correct proportions with alcohol and hexachlorophene, it can be an effective germicidal agent that will kill bacteria, spores, and even some viruses. The strong fumes given off by formalin or a solution containing formalin are irritating to respiratory passages.

The table of Common Chemical Disinfectants is again presented in this unit, figure 11-2. The unit on Microbial Control (Unit 8) should be reviewed.

SUMMARY

Cold or chemical sterilization kills pathogenic bacteria and in some cases will destroy nonpathogenic bacteria, spores, and viruses.

However, the effectiveness of chemical sterilization for actual sterile conditions is questionable. It should be considered as a method of disinfection. The medical assistant should remember that the term *sterilization* is not always accurate in this situation. Chemical sterilization is best used as a method of killing pathogens in medical asepsis.

All chemicals in use should be labeled and instructions for their use should be carefully read and understood *before* handling. Chemicals can be very caustic and result in damage to the tissues. They would NOT be used on an open wound.

SUGGESTED ACTIVITIES

- Using a hospital supply catalog, list some commercially prepared germicidal solutions together with their claims for effectiveness. Find at least five that claim to be effective against spores and viruses or fungi.

- Review sterile surgical asepsis and medical asepsis. Discuss where chemical sterilization fits into these two categories.

REVIEW

1. What does germicidal action mean?

2. Explain what is meant when it is said that disinfectant solutions are limited in their usage.

3. List two reasons for using chemical sterilization.

4. List three desired requirements of an effective disinfectant solution.

5. Why should all articles placed into chemical sterilization solutions be absolutely dry?

6. What does "caustic to tissues" mean?

7. What is the most widely used disinfectant? What strength is most effective?

8. What chemical is the standard for other germicides but is very caustic and most often mixed with some other chemical agent? What strength is most often used?

9. Which chemical will kill spores and viruses when mixed with alcohol and hexachlorophene but can be very irritating to respiratory passages?

10. Is chemical sterilization best used as a method of killing pathogens in medical or surgical asepsis? Would it be used on an open wound?

Unit 12 The Sterile Field

OBJECTIVES

After studying this unit, the student should be able to

- Set up a sterile field, using sterile technique.
- Explain and demonstrate the use of sterile pick-up forceps.
- State three ways how a sterile field can be contaminated.

The assistant must be able to set up and maintain a sterile field in order to assist the doctor with various surgically aseptic procedures.

In previous units, medical and surgical asepsis and how it is achieved have been discussed. Now, the medical assistant must learn how to set up a sterile field in a way that will not contaminate the sterile articles that have been made free of all living organisms through proper sterilization techniques. The skills discussed here must be practiced until the technique is correct. Cleanliness is not enough, sterility must be maintained. Remember, *surgical asepsis* is that procedure that protects internal tissues from destructive, infectious organisms. One of the medical assistant's responsibilities will be to help in the care of wounds or breaks in the skin.

Anything that touches a wound or a break in the skin must be sterile; just clean is not enough. Since hands cannot be sterilized, they must never touch sterile objects directly. Sterile gloves must be worn or sterile transfer forceps must be used when handling sterile objects.

THE STERILE FIELD

A dry, sterile towel is used to cover the tray, stand, or other area which is to be used for the sterile fields. Since the towel, itself, is sterile the medical assistant must handle it carefully to avoid contaminating the side upon which the sterile items are to be placed.

After opening the pack — keeping it away from the body while doing so — the medical assistant picks up the tip of the corner of the towel, withdraws the other hand and outside packing, and gently lets the towel unfold. She must be careful not to let the towel touch anything. Returning the other hand to another tip of the towel, she is then able to open the towel and lay it on the tray, again being very careful not to permit it to touch her uniform. Naturally, the side of the towel which rests on the tray will no longer be sterile; however, the side which makes up the sterile field will be sterile and is ready for the placement of sterile supplies and equipment. Leave a one-inch border (around the sterile field) free of any articles.

Never talk, cough, or sneeze over or near a sterile field. Airbone infection or droplets from the mouth contaminate the entire sterile field. Never bend directly over the setup, hair, dust, or other difficult to see contaminants may drop into the sterile field, contaminating it. This is one reason that a one-inch border around the inside edge of a sterile field is considered unsterile even though it has not been contaminated. All sterile articles are placed in the center of the setup, not on or near the edge.

Transfer of Sterile Objects

Sterile transfer or pick-up forceps are kept in a sterile container which contains a

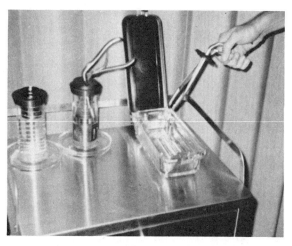

Fig. 12-1 Using sterile pick-up forceps.

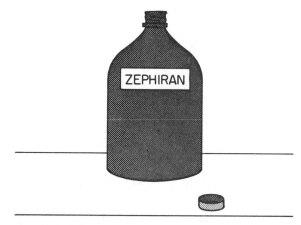

Fig. 12-2 When a cap is removed from a bottle containing a sterile solution, it is laid with the inside up.

very strong chemical that maintains the sterility of the forceps. When being used, the forceps must be carefully lifted out of the container without touching the outside rim of the container. Remember, some pathogens are airborne and articles left exposed to the air are contaminated. The forceps are always held so that the sterile end is never higher than the nonsterile or contaminated end (the handle), figure 12-1. If the forceps are not held correctly, the solution which is on the forceps will run up toward the handle, touch contaminated parts of the forceps, then run back down to the sterile end, thus contaminating the forceps.

The chemical solution in the forceps jar and container must be changed regularly in order to ensure its continued effectiveness.

Forceps are used to transfer sterile articles from one sterile setting to another. Therefore, the ends must remain sterile to avoid contamination of all articles. Gently tap the two prongs of the forceps together over the forceps jar to remove excess solution in order to avoid dripping the sterile solution onto the sterile field that is being prepared. Sterile objects that are made of paper or cloth do not remain sterile if they become wet.

When sterile articles are being removed from their sterile containers, great care must

be taken so the objects do not touch the outside of the container they are stored in. The outside of the container will be clean but not sterile and if sterile objects touch unsterile areas, they are contaminated. Covers are removed very carefully with one hand, held inside downward. The articles are removed with sterile forceps with the other hand. The cover is then replaced carefully.

When transferring sterile articles onto the sterile field that is covered with a dry, sterile towel, articles are dropped onto the field, never placed directly on it. The forceps must not touch the sterile setup.

Once a sterile article has left its container, it cannot be returned even if it has not been used. After it has been removed from the protective surroundings that maintained its sterility, technically it is unsterile due to air exposure. If it has not been used, it remains clean, but no longer sterile and must be sterilized again.

When pouring sterile solutions onto a sterile setup, never touch the container being poured from to the container on the sterile field. A two-inch space should be maintained at all times between the two containers.

When caps are removed from bottles that contain sterile solutions, they are inverted on the counter so that the inside rim does not

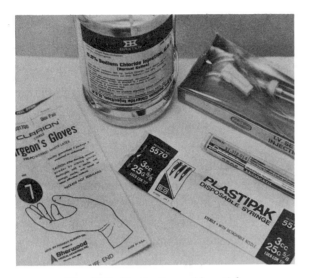

Fig. 12-3 Sterile disposable articles.

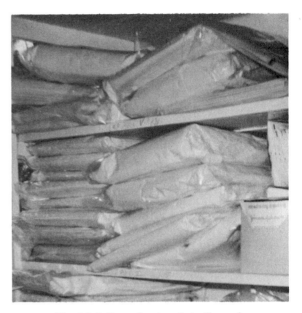

Fig. 12-4 Loosely stored sterile packs.

touch the contaminated counter of the cabinet. The fingers must not touch the rim either.

All sterile procedures and articles are handled above the waist. If an article is held below the waist, it automatically becomes contaminated.

When opening sterile packs, touch only the little tips of the wrap which were prefolded in the opposite direction for this pur-

pose. Disposable articles are usually packaged in a paper wrap that is especially designed to maintain sterility of the article inside. Open these packages as directed. Paper flaps are usually present on the package to avoid contamination of the articles inside. Follow the printed directions.

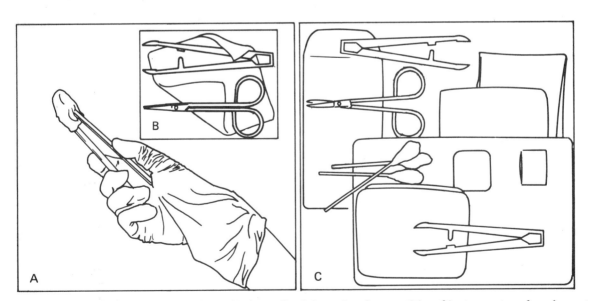

Fig. 12-5 The availability of disposable medical supplies is lessening the quantities of instruments and equipment which must be sterilized after each use. Disposable equipment shown includes: (A) examination gloves, (B) suture removal kit, (C) dressing tray.

Should a sterile article, object, or even an entire sterile setup become accidentally contaminated, it must be set aside for sterilization before it can be used again. The setup procedure must be repeated. If in doubt as to whether the sterility has been contaminated, do not take chances, set up a new sterile field. In the event the medical assistant sees the doctor contaminate the field, he must be told that he has contaminated the sterile field as he may not be aware that he has done so. Chances cannot be taken with a patient's life and wellbeing!

SUMMARY

Sterile technique must be used when setting up a sterile field. If a sterile field becomes contaminated in any way or if there is a question as to whether or not contamination has occurred, set up another sterile field.

Sterile forceps are used to transfer sterile objects from their containers to the sterile field. The outside of the containers are nonsterile and must not come into contact with the sterile field. Sterile gloves must be used in order to touch sterile articles. Forceps are used to set up a sterile field.

SUGGESTED ACTIVITIES

- Practice setting up a sterile field with a classmate watching very carefully to see that the sterile area is not contaminated.

- Practice opening sterile packs and disposable objects without contaminating the sterile objects inside.

- Practice using the transfer forceps in sterile technique.

- Practice pouring sterile solutions from their containers into a sterile glass or container on the sterile field.

REVIEW

Briefly answer the following questions.

1. What instrument is used to set up a sterile field without contaminating the sterile objects being placed on the field?

2. How are forceps held? Why?

3. How are lids or covers to sterile containers held while removing sterile supplies?

4. What area of a sterile field is not actually contaminated but is considered so?

5. Name two ways how a sterile field could be contaminated even though it is not touched.

6. If a can of cotton balls has been sterilized in the autoclave, why is the outside of the can considered unsterile?

7. Why is a sterile field contaminated by someone bending directly over it?

8. How does one treat sterile articles that were not used during a surgical aseptic procedure and are not dirty?

9. If a sterile solution wets a sterile setup, what effect does it have, if any, on the sterile field?

10. Why is the cap from a bottle of sterile solution laid upside-down on the table top while the solution is being poured?

11. How are sterile disposable articles opened?

12. What should you do if you see the doctor contaminate the sterile field?

Self-Evaluation Test 2

Choose the answers that best complete the following statements.

1. Some examples of one-celled plants are

   a. fungi.   c. bacteria.
   b. viruses.   d. rickettsiae.

2. The rod-shaped cells that are straight and slender or shaped like sausage are

   a. algae.   c. diplococci.
   b. bacilli.   d. flagella.

3. Bacteria that are able to move about or to twist and turn are

   a. rickettsiae.   c. spores.
   b. spirochetes.   d. cocci.

4. The only bacteria that is unable to form spores is the group classified as

   a. spiral-shaped.   c. spherical-shaped.
   b. rod-shaped.   d. anaerobic bacteria.

5. The primary purpose of microbial control is to

   a. prevent environmental pollution.
   b. kill all bacteria and other types of organisms that are found in our environment.
   c. prevent the spread of contagious and infectious diseases.
   d. maintain proper methods of medical and surgical asepsis.

6. All of the following methods except one will kill pathogenic organisms that are dangerous. Indicate the one method that does not kill pathogens.

   a. disinfection.   c. dry heat.
   b. autoclaving.   d. handwashing.

7. The most effective method of sterilization is

   a. dry heat.   c. disinfection.
   b. chemical sterilization.   d. moist heat under pressure.

8. When autoclaving, timing does not begin until

   a. the temperature reaches 93.3°C (200°F) and the pressure gauge reads 15 pounds pressure.
   b. the temperature reaches 121.1°C (250°F) and the pressure reaches 12 pounds per square inch.
   c. the temperature reaches 121.1°C (250°F) and the pressure reaches 15 pounds per square inch.
   d. ten minutes after the required temperature and pressure are reached.

9. The only type of sterilization that is guaranteed to kill all organisms, both pathogenic and nonpathogenic, is

   a. chemical sterilization with pure phenol.
   b. a hot air oven at 176.7°C (350°F) for one hour.
   c. temperatures that are maintained at below 0°C for at least 24 hours.
   d. temperatures above 121.1°C (250°F) at 15 lbs/sq. in. for 30 minutes.

10. The small office sterilizer works on the principle of

    a. a pressure cooker.   c. disinfection.
    b. boiling water.   d. hot air oven.

11. The sterilizer is used for sterilizing

    a. small, blunt instruments.   c. rubber and plastic equipment.
    b. small, sharp instruments.   d. large metal pans and containers.

12. The sterilizer will kill living organisms except

    a. fungi.   c. spirochetes.
    b. bacteria.   d. spore-forming organisms.

13. In order to sterilize equipment using the boiling method, the temperature which must be maintained throughout the timing process is

    a. 100°F (37.8°C).   c. 100°C.
    b. 212°C.   d. 250°F (121.1°C).

14. Chemical sterilization would be used in instances when

    a. time is not a factor.
    b. it is necessary to kill all organisms.
    c. the articles can be damaged by heat.
    d. all of the above.

15. The most widely used disinfecting solution is

    a. 99% alcohol.   c. hexachlorophene.
    b. 70% alcohol.   d. formalin.

16. In order to set up and maintain a sterile field, the medical assistant must know

    a. transfer techniques.
    b. surgical asepsis techniques.
    c. how microorganisms are transferred.
    d. all of the above.

17. If a sterile object has been removed from its protective surroundings but is not used, it is

    a. still sterile if placed back into the container.
    b. clean but not sterile and may be put back into the sterile container.
    c. clean but not sterile and must be sterilized again.
    d. contaminated and must be washed, dried, and sterilized again.

18. Any object that is introduced into an opening or break in the skin must be
    a. clean.
    b. medically aseptic.
    c. surgically aseptic.
    d. none of the above.

19. When a sterile setup is believed to have been contaminated
    a. ask the doctor if it is actually contaminated.
    b. remove the article that you suspect of being contaminated from the sterile field and replace it.
    c. consider the entire field contaminated and set up a new field with all sterile equipment.
    d. consider the expense and time involved and hope that the field was not actually contaminated.

20. In setting up a sterile field the assistant must use
    a. transfer forceps.
    b. her hands, being careful not to touch the sterile liquids.
    c. disposable gloves on her hands, being sure that they are clean, unused ones.
    d. sterile transfer forceps or sterile pick-up forceps.

Section 3
Treatments

Unit 13 Assisting with Minor Surgery

OBJECTIVES

After studying this unit, the student should be able to

- List the articles included on a minor surgery tray setup.
- State the medical assistant's responsibility in preparing the patient mentally and physically for minor surgery.
- Demonstrate the proper technique for a skin prep.

The patient who is to undergo minor surgery must be prepared mentally and physically for the procedure. The physician informs the patient of the surgery that is to be done and explains it thoroughly. The medical assistant offers reassurance and encouragement to the patient. She also gives any help she can in answering questions the patient might have but is reluctant to ask the physician.

PREPARING THE PATIENT

Specific positioning and draping of the patient will be determined by the kind of surgical procedure to be done. The medical assistant will prepare the patient; however, if in doubt about the way the patient is to be draped and/or positioned, she may check with the physician.

Besides meeting the patient's need for emotional support, positioning and draping, the assistant must prepare the skin for surgery. Hair is considered a source of contamination in some surgical procedures so the doctor may request that the area be shaved to prevent contamination of the internal tissues.

The Skin Prep

The procedure used to prepare the skin for surgery is referred to as the *skin prep*. The patient is covered by a lightweight bath blanket; this prevents chilling and is more comfortable for the patient during the skin prep. Also, it is easier for the assistant to handle than a sheet would be.

The skin prep involves shaving the hair and applying an antiseptic to reduce the number of microorganisms on the skin. (The skin cannot be completely sterilized; the cells would be destroyed in the process).

The assistant may use a disposable skin prep pack or she may have to prepare a tray with the necessary items. A prep tray should contain the following:

- Small sponge basin
- Several gauze sponges (4 x 4 inch squares)
- Disposable safety razor and blades
- Soapy antiseptic solution (such as Phisohex)
- Emesis basin (used for discarding gauze sponges)

A gooseneck lamp focused on the prep site will make the procedure safer for the patient and easier for the medical assistant as it will enable the medical assistant to see more clearly.

CAUTION: The area shaved must not be cut or nicked by the razor. Any cut or wound in the skin will allow pathogens to enter the body and cause infection. Report any cuts or abrasions to the doctor.

Soap the area before shaving, using the soapy solution and the gauze sponges. (Discard each sponge after use). After removing all hair from the skin surface, an antiseptic indicated by the doctor is applied to the skin. Apply the liquid to the skin in a circular motion *from the center of the site outward.* Do not rub back and forth over the same area. Sterile forceps and gauze sponges should be used to apply the skin antiseptic. Be sure to apply it to all of the skin surface being prepared.

The patient must not touch the area that has been prepared. If the assistant does the skin prep, she should cover the area with a sterile towel until such time as the doctor begins the surgery.

Before beginning the procedure, the doctor will drape the surgical site with additional

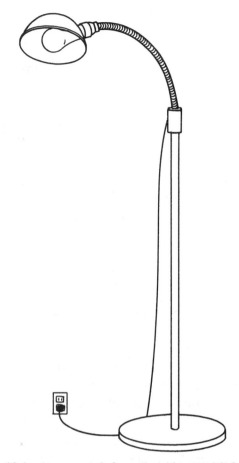

Fig. 13-1 **A gooseneck lamp provides good lighting for a skin prep.**

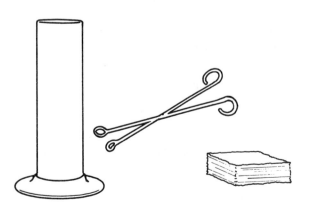

Fig. 13-2 **Sterile forceps container, forceps and sponges.**

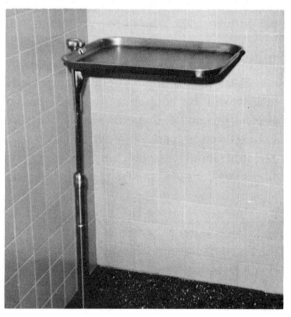

Fig. 13-3 **Mayo stand used for tray setups.**

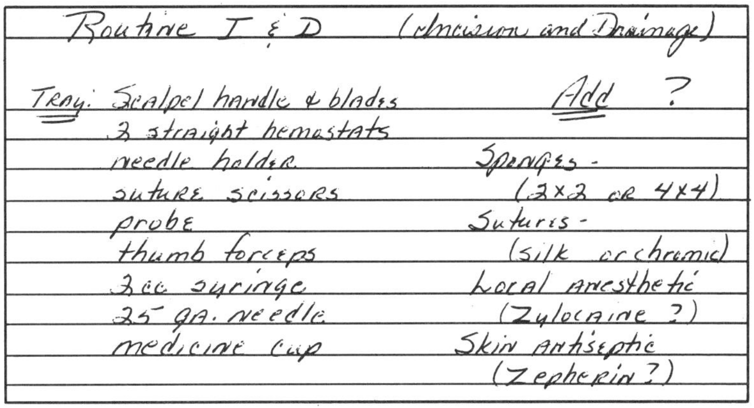
Routine I & D (Incision and Drainage)
Tray: Scalpel handle & blades — Add ?
3 straight hemostats
needle holder — Sponges -
suture scissors — (2x2 or 4x4)
probe — Sutures -
thumb forceps — (silk or chromic)
3cc syringe — Local anesthetic
25 ga. needle — (Zylocaine ?)
medicine cup — Skin antiseptic
(Zepherin ?)

Fig. 13-4 Sample file card for routine surgical procedure.

surgical (sterile) drapes and/or towels. Occasionally, the assistant may be asked to drape the surgical area. She must be careful not to contaminate any of the sterile drapes.

PREPARING THE TREATMENT ROOM

A minor surgery tray is set up on a Mayo stand near the patient and convenient to the doctor. This is a sterile setup and contains the following articles.

- Scapel handle and blades
- Hemostats (curved or straight)
- Needle holder
- Needles and suture materials (catgut or silk)
- Suture scissors
- Thumb forceps
- Probe
- Sponges (gauze squares)
- Container for local anesthetic solution
- Syringes and needles
- Hand towel
- Dressings

Remember, *all articles must be sterile.* The tray may be prepared, wrapped in a pack, and then sterilized or set up using sterile articles. Asepsis technique was discussed in the previous unit; it should be reviewed, if necessary.

In addition to the minor surgery tray or setup – which will vary according to the doctor's preference and the particular procedure – packs will need to be prepared containing (1) sterile gown, (2) sterile gloves and, (3) surgical masks. These are available in disposable packages which are frequently used in doctor's offices. The assistant must set up and open packs for the doctor regardless of the type of packs used.

It is wise to keep a small file containing lists of instruments, solutions, sutures, etc. that the physician will use for each surgical procedure. This system saves time and avoids the need to ask the physician what he will need each time a routine procedure is done. Examine the illustration shown in figure 13-4.

ASSISTING THE PHYSICIAN

After preparing the patient and the treatment room, the medical assistant stands ready to lend reassurance to the patient and to hand the doctor any additional materials he may need. Occasionally, he may ask her to scrub and help him in the surgical field. This means that the assistant must remove all jewelry such as rings and wristwatch, scrub her hands carefully with a surgical scrub brush and soap, dry her hands on a sterile towel, and put on sterile gloves. She must be extremely careful to avoid any contamination with any object and keep the operative area sterile at all times. Any break in technique must be relayed to the doctor.

The doctor will always administer the anesthesia. It will usually be a local anesthetic unless a group of physicians are working together in an office which has extensive facilities for surgery and a qualified anesthesiologist (doctor who specializes in giving anesthesia).

Drugs usually given for local anesthesia are Procaine (Novocaine) and Lidocaine (Xylocaine).

- Procaine or Novocaine is used in 2% solution or less (usually 1/2%). It is the least toxic of the local anesthetics. It may be given subcutaneously, intramuscularly, intravenously, or by spinal injection.

If the patient's skin becomes flushed or his pulse increases, he may be hypersensitive to the drug. The assistant would bring this to the doctor's attention if it should occur, although, usually, the doctor has questioned the patient about any known allergies to drugs and other substances.

- Lidocaine or Xylocaine may be given by injection or topically. It lasts longer than procaine. It tends to spread beyond the site of the injection.

Usually, Procaine is used. The medical assistant must be sure that the materials the doctor would need in preparing for the injection of the anesthetic are on hand: sterile syringes and needles, sterile sponges, sterile medicine glasses, and a flask of sterile procaine solution (often 1/2% strength). The physician will pour the amount needed into the sterile glass and withdraw some of the procaine with a syringe. Then, using a small-gauge needle a small amount of the anesthetic is injected into the skin, initially. A larger needle will be used to inject the anesthetic deeper into the tissues.

When the procedure is finished and sterile dressings have been applied to the wound, the patient is helped off the table and into a more comfortable position.

CAUTION: Patients are not to be left alone after any surgical procedure until the assistant is absolutely certain that there is no danger of the patient fainting or falling. Delayed reactions to treatment sometimes occur.

The assistant also checks with the patient to be certain that all of the doctor's postoperative (after surgery) instructions are clearly understood.

After the assistant has cared for all of the patient's needs, she must clean up all equipment used in the procedure and prepare the room for the next patient.

SUMMARY

When assisting with minor surgery, the assistant must know how to organize the treatment room with the necessary equipment and articles. She must also assist with the preparation of the patient by reassuring the patient and answering any questions he might have about the procedure. The assistant will prepare the skin for surgery (skin prep) as indicated by the doctor. She will assist the doctor during minor surgery procedures by supplying the doctor with any additional articles or instruments he might need during the procedure. Occasionally, the assistant may be required to scrub and assist in the sterile field.

After the procedure is completed, the patient must not be left alone until there is no danger of the patient fainting or falling. The assistant must make sure the patient understands the doctor's postoperative instructions. The assistant will clean the treatment room and make it ready for the next patient. The assistant will also clean all the equipment used and return it to its proper place.

SUGGESTED ACTIVITIES

- Role play preparing for minor surgery. Have class members evaluate the activity and discuss it.
- Name three common minor surgical techniques. Make a list of the items necessary for these procedures.
- Prepare a setup for one of the procedures listed in the unit. Have a classmate check the technique used.
- Under guidance and observation of the instructor, practice performing a surgical scrub and putting on sterile surgical gloves.
- Learn the names of the more common surgical instruments used in minor surgery. Be able to identify each instrument by name and function.

REVIEW

A. Answer the questions in the space provided.

1. List the articles included on a minor surgery tray setup.

2. List the articles to be included on a skin prep tray.

3. Explain the correct procedure for performing a skin prep.

4. Name four responsibilities of the medical assistant AFTER minor surgery has been completed.

5. Name two ways how the medical assistant can prepare the patient mentally for minor surgery.

B. Select the correct word from Column II to describe the appropriate item in Column I. Place the correct *word* in the blank preceding the item.

<u>Column I</u>   <u>Column II</u>

1. _____ The area that is prepared   Postoperative
                            for a surgical procedure.   Sponges

2. _____ Small square gauze dressings.   Surgical site

3. _____ Means after surgery or surgical   Surgical drapes
                            procedures.   Preoperative
                                                                                      Skin prep
4. _____ A procedure that prepares the
                            skin before a surgical procedure.

5. _____ Sterile pieces of cloth or paper
                            used to surround the surgical
                            site.

C. Read each statement of responsibility carefully. After each responsibility, place the word *physician* or *assistant* on the line, *then explain your answer* in the space provided.

1. Informs the patient of the type of surgery that
   is to be done and explain it thoroughly.   _____

2. Positions and drapes the patient for minor
   surgery.   _____

3. Does the skin prep before surgery.   _____

4. Prepares the packs to be used during the surgery.   _____

5. Decides what instruments and equipment should
   be placed in the packs.   _____

6. Keeps a file of instruments and equipment listing certain setups for routine minor surgical procedures.   _____

D. Select the correct answer(s).

1. Skin prep trays used to shave a patient before a surgical procedure may be

   a. disposable.
   b. prepared by the assistant.
   c. set up by the physician.
   d. omitted entirely.

2. The assistant's responsibilities in actually assisting during the surgical procedure is limited to

   a. reassuring the patient.
   b. adding additional supplies to the setup.
   c. being ready to scrub in order to assist in the sterile field, if necessary.
   d. all of the above.

3. Which of the following statements are true?

   a. The medical assistant must be sure that all of the materials the doctor needs for anesthetic injection are on hand.
   b. Lidocaine or Xylocaine may be given by injection or topically.
   c. Procaine is the least toxic of the local anesthetics.
   d. If the patient's skin becomes flushed or his pulse increases, he may be hypersensitive to the drug.

Unit 14 Removal of Foreign Objects

OBJECTIVES

After studying this unit, the student should be able to

- State the rules for a medical assistant to follow when removing foreign objects from the eye, ear, nose, and skin.

- Explain how to remove an insect from the ear.

- Identify the medical assistant's responsibility in specifically stated cases involving removal of foreign objects.

Foreign objects often become caught in body tissues such as the skin, eyes, ears, and nostrils. Patients with this kind of problem are frequently found in a physician's office. This unit will review usual office procedures involved in cases of this kind.

PATIENT PREPARATION

This will depend upon what the foreign object is and where it is located. However, one of the first things to remember is that the patient will be frightened and anxious. Taking a few moments to calm and reassure the patient will make the patient feel much better and will also make dealing with that person much easier. Adults may be asked to lie down on the examiner's table or sit in a chair in the examiner's room. Adults will usually respond to verbal reassurances much better than children. If the patient is a child (as is often the case with foreign objects) reassure the parent and ask him or her to hold and reassure the child.

Sometimes it is necessary to restrain small children by wrapping them securely in a sheet or lightweight blanket; the parent or another person may hold the head firmly to prevent the child from thrashing around while the object is being removed.

FOREIGN OBJECTS IN THE SKIN

Any foreign object that has entered the skin should only be removed by the doctor. Sterile technique is necessary in order to prevent severe infections at the point of entry.

Foreign objects most often found in the skin are glass, splinters of wood, steel, and occasionally pieces of rock or stone. All of these objects are potentially dangerous and should be removed as soon as possible.

The physician will need a setup similar to that used for minor surgery. The assistant prepares the treatment room in much the same way, being sure to check with the doctor for any additional equipment that might be needed. After preparing the patient and the treatment room, the assistant helps during the procedure unless otherwise instructed by the physician.

FOREIGN OBJECTS IN THE EYE

The assistant should NEVER attempt to remove any foreign body embedded in the eyeball. If the object is causing intense pain and discomfort, the medical assistant should have the patient lie down. If the doctor cannot be reached immediately, the medical assistant may *gently and lightly* apply cold sterile compresses to the affected eye until he is contacted.

Under no circumstances should the assistant probe the eye with any instrument or object.

Dust, cinders, insects, and many other objects may become lodged in the eye. The object may be underneath the eyelid, embedded in the eyelid, or even lodged in the eyeball itself. The safest thing to do is to cover the eye gently, to prevent any further damage by movement; apply a cold compress, and get the doctor as quickly as possible.

Sometimes, the physician may train the medical assistant to remove a foreign body, such as a speck of dirt, from the eye. If she has been trained and has permission, she may proceed with care. The speck must be visible; it may be necessary to evert the eyelid, figure 14-1. Remove the object with a cotton-tipped applicator which has been moistened with sterile water or normal saline. The speck is removed by gentle swabbing of the moist applicator. Again, there must be prior permission of the physician before the medical assistant would remove foreign objects from the eye. Under *no* circumstances would she remove an object which is embedded, or is on the *cornea* of the eye. (The eyeball has three coats, the sclera, cornea, and retina. The cornea is the translucent bulge that comes forth slightly in the middle, front part of the eyeball.)

If a chemical should get in the eye, the eye should be immediately flushed with large amounts of lukewarm water; this should be done quickly but gently. The flow of water should be directed from the inner angle (near the nose) to the outer angle (toward the ear). Then the eye should be covered with a large sterile gauze sponge until the doctor can see it.

FOREIGN OBJECTS IN THE EAR

Children often put foreign objects in their ears. Peas, beads, cotton or anything else to which the child has access may eventually find its way into one or both ears!

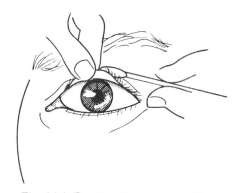

Fig. 14-1 Everting the upper eyelid.

If the object is far down into the ear canal, the assistant should not attempt to remove it as it may merely move farther down. The physician must see these patients. If it is located just within the ear and can be easily removed without injury, the assistant may use a cotton-moistened applicator to remove it.

If the foreign object is an insect, the assistant may instill a few drops of warm oil, such as mineral oil. The oil causes the insect to suffocate. This stops the movement which was the cause for the patient's severe discomfort. When the insect is dead, the oil and insect can be easily removed from the ear with the aid of a cotton-tipped swab. CAUTION: Never place oil or any liquid in a patient's ear that contains an object other than an insect! The liquid could make a foreign body, such as a dry bean or bead, swell thus causing even more discomfort and pain. This would also make the removal of the object more difficult.

FOREIGN OBJECTS IN THE NOSE

Again, this situation is most often found in children who have intentionally put some foreign object up the nose. The objects are of the same variety that children are prone to stuff into their ears.

If the object is visible and may be removed without the aid of instruments (such as by gently squeezing the nostrils *above* the foreign body) the assistant may try to remove it. If however, it is embedded deeply in the nasal passage, the doctor must remove the object. As previously mentioned, the medical assistant must be sure *she has the physician's permission, beforehand, to perform any office procedure at which he is not present,* however minor it may be.

GENERAL RULES

General rules to follow when removing foreign objects are:

- Never attempt to remove foreign objects from the eye. The physician must do this. Cold compresses to relieve the discomfort and minimize eye movements may be used until the doctor can treat the patient.

- In the event the patient has chemical solution in the eye, the eye should be immediately flushed with water before covering it with the cold compress and calling the doctor.

- The doctor will remove objects which are in the ear canal. Those objects which are just within the ear or nose and can be seen may be removed if no instruments are required and the assistant has prior permission.

- Foreign objects embedded in the skin are to be removed by the doctor only. The assistant may assist the physician in the procedure.

SUMMARY

It is very important for the medical assistant to know what foreign objects she may attempt to remove and what objects are to be removed by the doctor only. Objects in the eyes or those which have entered the skin should *not* be removed by the assistant.

Foreign objects in the ear or nose, which can be removed without using any type of instrument may be removed by the assistant if she has permission to do so. Insects which have entered the ear may first be killed by using warm oil, such as mineral oil, and then removed with a cotton-tipped swab. Liquids are never applied to foreign objects other than insects that might be in the ear or nose. The liquid may cause swelling of the object thus making it more painful and more difficult for the doctor to remove.

SUGGESTED ACTIVITIES.

- Discuss some familiar cases where foreign objects have been removed from patients.

- Discuss possible reactions of the medical assistant in the following cases:

  a. A fisherman has a fishhook embedded in his hand. He asks the assistant to remove it for him since he does not have time to wait for the doctor.

  b. A child has packed his ear with soft cooked peas.

  c. A lady needs immediate relief because an insect is caught in her nose.

REVIEW

A. Answer the following questions.

   1. Explain the procedure for removing an insect from a patient's ear.

2. List the rules that a medical assistant must follow when removing foreign objects from the (1) eye (2) ear and nose and (3) skin.

3. Why is it important for the medical assistant to take a few minutes to calm and reassure the patient who has a foreign object which needs to be removed?

4. Other than to remove an insect, why must oil or liquid NEVER be -used to remove a foreign object from a patient's ear or nose?

B. Select the answer that best describes the medical assistant's responsibility in the following cases.

1. A young woman has come to the office complaining of "burning eyes" after accidentally spraying hair spray in her eyes.

   a. Have her sit down and wait until the doctor can see her.
   b. Have her lie down and apply cold compresses to her eyes.
   c. Ask the patient what was in the spray so you can call the doctor who is out.
   d. Flush the eyes carefully with lukewarm water and cover them with cold compresses until the doctor can see her.

2. A man comes into the office with a fish fin embedded in his finger. Part of the fin is sticking out of the skin but not far enough to grasp and pull. The doctor is in.

   a. Ask the man to wait until the doctor can see him.
   b. Explain the situation to the doctor and insist that the man be seen immediately.
   c. Reassure the man, inform the doctor, and carry out his instructions.
   d. Try to remove the fin with surgical tweezers.

3. A child has a small dried pea in his ear and is crying and fighting to get away from his mother. The doctor is in.

   a. Reassure the mother and child, wrap the child in a sheet, and ask the mother to hold his head while you look to see if the bean can be removed without difficulty.
   b. Flush the ear with lukewarm water and see if the pea floats out.
   c. Remove the pea with a pair of rubber-tipped forceps.
   d. Wrap the child securely, have the mother hold him, and instill warm mineral oil into the ear.

4. A woman has an insect crawling around inside her ear. It is extremely painful and she is very apprehensive and in great distress. The doctor is out.

   a. Apply cold compresses and have her wait until the doctor returns. Reassure and calm her.
   b. Instill tepid water into the ear and float the insect out.
   c. Send her to the hospital where the doctor is.
   d. Drop warm mineral oil into the ear to suffocate the insect.

5. A young man has some unidentified object in his eye that is causing him much pain and discomfort. The doctor is out.

   a. Inspect the eye to determine what the object is. If you can't see anything, have him wait until the doctor returns.
   b. Wash the eye out with lukewarm water and send him to the hospital emergency room.
   c. Cover the eye with cold compresses, tell him not to move his eye under the compresses, and contact the doctor.
   d. Inspect the eye to determine what the object is. If you can find the object, remove it.

Unit 15 Dressings and Bandages

OBJECTIVES

After completing this unit, the student should be able to

- Differentiate between a dressing and bandage.
- List four purposes of bandages and give an example of situations where each may be used.
- Name two types of dressings and tell when each is used.
- Set up a dressing tray with necessary items.
- Demonstrate ability to apply a dressing and a bandage.

There are different kinds of dressings and bandages. The medical assistant must know when and where they are to be used.

DRESSINGS

A *dressing* is a covering used to protect an open wound. The kind of dressing used will depend upon the wound it is designed to protect. There are several kinds of wounds such as cuts, burns, abrasions (the scraping away of the skin surface) and eruptions. If the wound is not draining it is said to be a clean wound; a dry, sterile dressing is applied. If the wound is draining, either a dry dressing (heavily padded to absorb the drainage) or a wet dressing is applied. When a wet dressing is indicated, sterile solution and materials are necessary. Occasionally, the doctor will insert a small rubber or plastic tube into a draining wound and then cover it with either dry or wet dressings.

If the wound is a surgical wound, it will be covered with sterile, dry dressings; these dressings are most often made of gauze. They are secured by adhesive or cellophane tape. If the patient is sensitive to adhesive tape, cellophane tape is used. Sometimes a dressing called *telfa* is placed next to the wound to prevent the dressing from sticking to the wound. When a dressing sticks to a wound, its removal is difficult and painful. Each physician will choose the type of dressings he prefers. The assistant will prepare the dressing cart or tray and assist the doctor in applying the dressing, if he desires.

A dressing tray or cart must contain the following sterile materials:

- Sterile pickup forceps and jar
- Sterile dressing forceps and/or sterile hemostats
- Medications such as solutions to cleanse the wound
- Bandage scissors
- Tape used to secure the dressing

It is the duty of the medical assistant to keep the dressing tray well supplied with sterile and clean equipment. Everything should be kept in readiness for immediate use.

Asepsis is practiced at all times by the doctor and the assistant during a dressing change or application. All soiled dressings are discarded into a basin close to the treatment table, within reach of the doctor. Any dressings that are removed from a wound and anything else that comes in contact with a wound is contaminated.

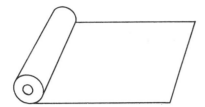

Fig. 15-1 Roller bandage.

When removing a dressing, always pull the *skin* away from the tape, not the tape away from the skin. This should be done quickly. The tape should always be removed in the direction of the wound; pulling tape away from the wound may pull the wound open again.

BANDAGES

Bandages are applications of cloth (or plaster of paris in the case of a cast) that serve several purposes. A bandage may be used to hold a dressing in place over a wound or it may be used to apply pressure to prevent swelling or hemorrhage (bleeding). It may also be used to immobilize (prevent freedom of movement) an injured part of the body as in splints used with fractures until the fracture can be reduced (or set). Bandages can also be used to protect or support an injured part of the body. Slings are an example of this kind of bandage.

Varieties

There are several varieties of bandages that are commonly used in the doctor's office. Roller bandage made of gauze is most often used. It comes in several widths. The width used depends upon what kind of bandage is needed and the part of the body where it is to be applied. Roller gauze can be obtained in widths from ½ inch to 4 inches and also in varying lengths (usually 10 yards). The roller gauze bandage restricts movement a great deal.

Another type of roller bandage is made of elastic material that will stretch and expand if edema or swelling occurs. The elastic-type bandage also permits a limited amount of movement.

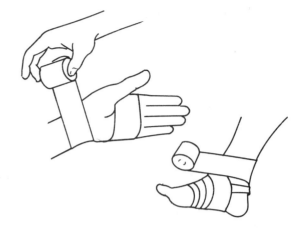

Fig. 15-2 Figure-of-eight bandages.

Roller bandages may be applied in many different ways. A circular bandage may be applied in order to hold a dressing in place. This might be used around a small dressing on the arm or leg. If the dressing is large, it may be secured with an ascending spiral bandage. (This is a bandage going upward). Figure-of-eight bandages are used on hands, feet, ankles, and elbows. The bandage is always adapted to the purpose of the bandage as well as to the part of the body being bandaged.

If the bandage is a cast made of plaster of paris, it must be applied by the doctor; the medical assistant will be called upon to assist. Plaster of paris sets very rapidly and hardens when exposed to air so work must be done rapidly and efficiently. Casts are used to immobilize injured extremities or other movable parts of the body.

Triangular bandages are most often used as slings to support an injured arm, elbow, shoulder, or hand. A sling will support the arm and hand and will restrict movement as well. Triangular bandages may be made from a square, folded diagonally, figure 15-3.

The application of bandages is very important. Skin surfaces should never touch. For example, the toes of the foot should not be bandaged together; gauze should be placed between the toe's skin surfaces before the bandage is applied to hold the dressing in place.

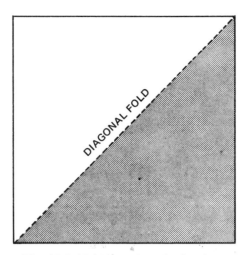

Fig. 15-3 Making a triangular bandage.

When roller bandages are used, the bandage must be applied without wrinkles and in a manner that will hold the dressing in place without impeding circulation. A bandage should not be so tight as to be uncomfortable to the patient but should be tight enough to serve its purpose.

Roller bandages are always applied starting with the inside of the roll facing the assistant. It is anchored firmly by two or three turns around the dressing and then applied smoothly. If it is to be a spiral bandage, the edges will overlap.

SUMMARY

Dressings are coverings used to protect open wounds. They may be dry or wet but are always sterile. Dressings help to prevent infection of the wound and also help to prevent the spreading of infection if the wound is draining.

Bandages are used to hold dressings in place, apply pressure, immobilize an injured area, or protect and support an injury. The bandage is always adapted to the purpose it is intended to serve, as well as to the area where it is to be applied.

SUGGESTED ACTIVITIES

- Using a classmate as the patient, practice applying sterile dressings. Use appropriate bandages to hold the dressings in place. Ask the instructor to evaluate the aseptic technique and also the competency of the activity.

- Practice applying bandages to a foot, wrist, and arm.

- Invite a representative from the local Red Cross chapter to demonstrate the types of bandaging used in emergency situations.

- Make arrangements for the class to participate in a Red Cross multimedia course. (This can be completed in one day if prearranged with the local Red Cross chapter.)

REVIEW

A. Define the following terms.

1. Dressing

2. Bandage

B. Beside each statement, place the word *dressing* or *bandage.* Be sure to read the statement carefully before deciding which word best applies to that statement.

1. A _____ is used to support a sprained elbow.

2. A _____ is used to cover and protect a draining wound.

3. A _____ is used to immobilize a fractured ankle.

4. A _____ is used to protect an incision after surgery.

5. A _____ is used to prevent the spread of infection from a draining wound.

6. A _____ is used to secure a sterile covering for an injury.

7. A _____ may serve several different purposes such as holding a dressing in place and applying pressure to an injured area.

C. Answer the following questions.

1. Name the items which should be contained on a dressing tray.

2. Name the four purposes of bandages and give an example of each.

3. Name two types of dressings and give an example of when each is used.

4. Roller bandages may be applied in many different ways; name two of them.

5. Both types of dressings are applied with aseptic technique. Why?

Unit 16 Hot and Cold Applications

OBJECTIVES

After completing this unit, the student should be able to

- Demonstrate how to set up a tray for application of warm, moist, sterile compresses.
- Identify what treatments and techniques would be done in specifically stated situations.
- Describe how heat and cold affect local areas.

The medical assistant must be familiar with the application of heat and cold in a way that is safe and beneficial to the patient. She must be familiar with the principles of application of heat and cold and the expected results of the treatment. The skin has nerve endings (receptors) which receive the heat or cold stimulation. They transmit the sensation to the underlying tissues, figure 16-1.

HEAT APPLICATIONS

When heat is applied to the body, an excess of blood is concentrated in the area of ap-

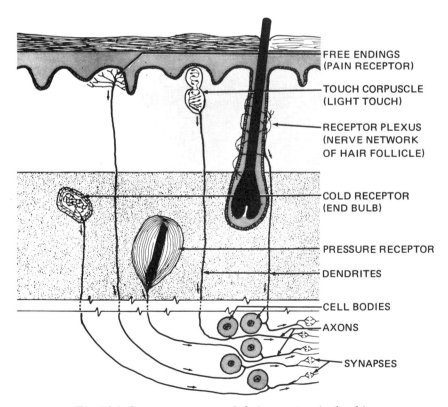

Fig. 16-1 Sensory neurons and their receptors in the skin.

(From Memmler, R. and Rada D. *The Human Body and Disease.* Philadelphia: Lippincott, 1970)

plication. Heat causes blood vessels to dilate. This results in increased circulation in the area.

The purpose of applying heat is to relieve inflammation and congestion. Heat also relaxes muscles, tendons, and ligaments.

Dry Heat

The application of dry heat is relatively easy; a heating pad or a hot water bottle will serve this purpose. Sometimes a heat lamp is used.

If an electric heating pad is used, be very careful not to allow the heating pad to become wet or to use any metal pins in it. Be sure there is at least one thickness of towel between the pad and the patient's skin. The physician will indicate the length of time the heat application is to be given.

If a hot water bottle is used, it should be wrapped in two thicknesses of towel before being placed on the patient's body. The bag is filled with water (49° to 52°C or 120° to 125°F). The hot-water bag should be filled 1/3 to 1/2 full. The excess air is expelled by placing the bag on a flat surface and holding the neck of the bag upright until the water reaches the neck, figure 16-2. The bag is then folded at the neck and closed by anchoring the ends. Some hot-water bottles simply have a top which may be screwed on after the air has been expelled. Be sure to dry off any excess water on the outside before wrapping it in the towel or cover.

Moist Heat

Moist heat is applied by using compresses. These compresses are usually 2 x 2 inch or 4 x 4 inch gauze squares. Moist heat is usually more beneficial than dry heat as moisture increases the effectiveness of heat. Moist heat is often used to localize infection and aid drainage.

Any application of moist heat must be carried out very carefully so as not to burn tis-

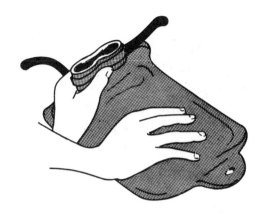

Fig. 16-2 Force air out of hot water bottle.

sues. If the area where the compresses are to be applied has an open wound or any drainage, *sterile* compresses must be used. If drainage is present, each compress must be carefully discarded after application and a sterile compress applied in its place. If there is no drainage, the same, clean compress may be used again.

To apply hot, moist compresses, the assistant needs gauze sponges (usually 4 x 4 inches) a hotplate, a basin, and the solution; normal saline or water is frequently used. Two pairs of forceps are used to wring out excess moisture from the compress before applying it to the patient's skin. The preferred solution is heated in a small basin until slightly warmer than skin temperature, not to exceed 115°F (which is about 46°C). The gauze sponges are placed in the solution and then wrung out, using two pairs of forceps. The compresses are straightened and laid gently on the area *without allowing the forceps to touch the skin.* Besides being likely to burn the patient's skin, touching it would contaminate the forceps.

The compresses will cool quickly once they are removed from the solution so they must be applied quickly and efficiently. The compresses must be replaced as they cool;

this procedure is repeated for 10 or 15 minutes unless the doctor specifies a longer treatment.

If the area being treated has a break in the skin or a wound of any type, the applications must be sterile. Aseptic technique is observed throughout the treatment. Any surface that touches a draining wound becomes contaminated so; (1) watch the forceps and (2) throw away all compresses after they have touched the wound.

COLD APPLICATIONS

The application of cold to the body surface contracts blood vessels. This action reduces inflammation, relieves congestion, reduces swelling and discoloration, relieves heat, and delays the formation of *purulent drainage* (pus).

The application of cold is often used as a treatment for burns, strains and sprains, or trauma resulting from a hard blow. Trauma may cause edema and discoloration.

Dry Cold

Cold may be applied to the body by filling an ice bag with crushed ice, checking it carefully for leaks, and wrapping it in a towel before applying it to the affected area. Single-use cold packs are also available.

Leaving cold compresses on a patient for too long can result in discomfort and injuries similar to the ones resulting from heat applications which have been applied for too long. No moisture should be allowed to accumulate on the patient's skin as it can be very uncomfortable. The assistant should check to be sure the area of the skin is kept dry.

Moist Cold

The same rules apply to moist cold applications as to moist hot compresses. If the area to be treated has an open wound or is draining, the procedure calls for aseptic technique. The compresses must be sterile and the

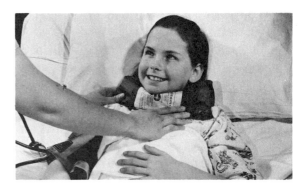

Fig. 16-3 A single-use cold pack.

contaminated gauze sponges discarded after each application. Clean technique will be sufficient if there is no open wound or drainage.

The solution used for moist cold compresses may be refrigerated before use. If the treatment is to be maintained for 10 to 15 minutes, the compresses must be changed frequently with small amounts of cold solution being added each time.

If it is not a sterile procedure, the initial compress may be applied and then an icebag placed over the wet compress. However, since the heat of the body will dry the compress fairly rapidly, it must be soaked again at frequent intervals.

Care should be taken to see that the patient does not become damp and chilled during the treatment. Check with the patient often to see if a lightweight blanket may be needed. Be sure that the patient is comfortable.

SUMMARY

When heat is applied to the body, the blood vessels in that area dilate. This action causes an increase in the flow of blood to the area, resulting in a relaxation of muscles, tendons, and ligaments. Heat also relieves inflammation and congestion.

Heat may be used as a treatment by applying it with or without moisture. Moisture increases the effectiveness of heat. Hot applications may be applied in either a sterile or unsterile manner; sterile applications are always indicated if the area being treated has an open wound.

When cold is applied, blood vessels constrict. This decreases circulation and blood flow. The results are reduction of inflammation, relief of congestion, reduction of edema and discoloration. Also, the production of purulent drainage is decreased. Cold may also be applied dry or wet and in a sterile or nonsterile manner.

Extreme care should be used when applying either hot or cold applications. The patient should be checked frequently to avoid burning or chilling.

SUGGESTED ACTIVITIES

- Set up a tray to be used for applying warm, moist, sterile compresses.
- Using sterile technique, practice applying warm, moist compresses to the inner arm of a classmate. Have her check your technique then exchange places.
- Apply cold, moist compresses to the back of the neck of a classmate. Did she feel chilled? What would a medical assistant do to avoid this sensation?

REVIEW

A. Select the answer that best completes the following statements.

1. When cold is applied to body surface
   a. the blood vessels dilate and circulation is decreased.
   b. the blood vessels constrict and circulation is decreased.
   c. the blood vessels dilate and circulation is increased.
   d. the blood vessels constrict and circulation is increased.

2. Cold is usually applied to the body for the purpose of
   a. muscle, tendon, and ligament relaxation.
   b. reduction of edema and discoloration.
   c. causing pus formation to be speeded up.
   d. speeding up the process of inflammation.

3. Heat may be applied to the body for the purpose of
   a. reduction of discoloration and edema.
   b. speeding up the process of pus formation.
   c. slowing down the inflammation process.
   d. none of the above.

B. Indicate whether hot or cold treatments would be indicated in the following cases and if sterile or nonsterile technique would be used.

	Treatment	Technique
1. A bruise caused by a baseball bat	_____	_____
2. A strained back muscle	_____	_____
3. A swelling cut from a fall	_____	_____
4. An insect sting	_____	_____
5. An infected surgical wound	_____	_____

Unit 17 Irrigations

OBJECTIVES

After completing this unit, the student should be able to

- List items required for eye and ear irrigations.
- Give reasons for taking specific precautions in irrigations.
- Demonstrate ability to irrigate the specified body cavity.
- Recognize and identify principles underlying each irrigation.

Irrigations are treatments that flush away particles or irritating matter from sensitive tissues. The solutions used will depend upon the area being irrigated as well as the solution preferred by the doctor.

All treatments are done only upon a physician's order and are carefully charted upon the patient's record. The results of the treatment should accompany the recording of the treatment as well as the time, date, and name of the person administering the treatment.

EYE IRRIGATIONS

The medical assistant should be familiar enough with eye structures to safely irrigate the eyes, figure 17-1.

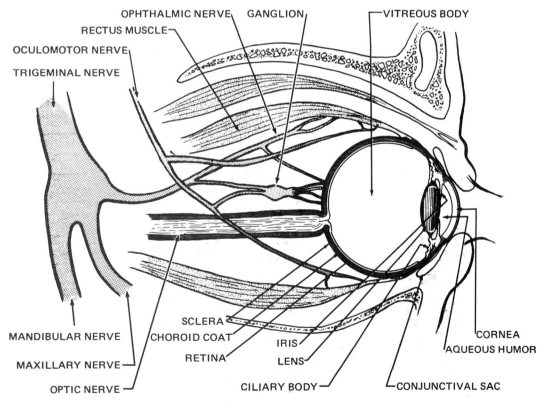

OPHTHALMIC NERVE GANGLION VITREOUS BODY
RECTUS MUSCLE
OCULOMOTOR NERVE
TRIGEMINAL NERVE

MANDIBULAR NERVE
MAXILLARY NERVE
OPTIC NERVE

SCLERA
CHOROID COAT
RETINA

IRIS
LENS
CILIARY BODY

CORNEA
AQUEOUS HUMOR
CONJUNCTIVAL SAC

Fig. 17-1 Structures of the eye.
(From Memmler, R. and Rada D. *The Human Body in Health and Disease.* Philadelphia: Lippincott, 1970)

The eye is irrigated (1) to cleanse and wash away foreign particles and (2) to alleviate pain and discomfort. The basic equipment used is a tray with the following equipment.

- A small sterile basin (to contain the irrigating solution)
- The solution to be used at 105°-115°F (40° - 46.1°C). *Do NOT EXCEED this temperature.*
- A sterile bulb syringe or an asepto syringe with a rubber tip (for irrigating the eye)
- A kidney-shaped emesis basin (for return flow)
- Sterile cotton balls or gauze sponges (for wiping)
- A towel (to place under the emesis basin)

Procedure

Gather all equipment and explain the procedure to the patient. If both eyes are to be irrigated, separate setups are needed to prevent crosscontamination.

The patient is placed in a comfortable position on the treatment table with the head slightly turned toward the medical assistant. The medical assistant works from the affected side, that is, the side that is being treated. For example, if the right eye is to be irrigated, the patient's head is turned toward the assistant, and she is at his right side.

The medical assistant proceeds in the following way.

1. Place the towel next to the face; set the emesis basin on the towel next to the cheek so that the irrigating solution will run into the basin. The patient may hold the basin.

2. Rest the hand that is holding the syringe on the bridge of the patient's nose, in order to prevent injury to the patient caused by sudden movement. A rubber tip on the irrigating syringe is an added

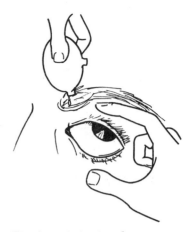

Fig. 17-2 Irrigating the eye.

safety measure to insure that the patient is not injured.

3. Dispel a small amount of the solution from the bulb (the solution in the very tip of the bulb becomes cold very quickly). Hold the patient's eye open gently by separating the lids with the index finger and thumb. Ask the patient to look up if possible. Slowly allow the warm solution to run from the inside corner of the eye to the outside corner. CAUTION: Be on guard for sudden movement from the patient when he feels the solution in his eye.

4. When all of the solution has been used in the irrigation procedure, gently remove the emesis basin and carefully wipe excess moisture from the patient's outer lids. Wipe from the inner to the outer side. Apply a dressing if ordered. Remember, *O.D.* means right eye and *O.S.* means left eye. The abbreviation, *O.U.* refers to both eyes. Charting must be accurate and descriptive of the results (relief, smarting, nature of return flow, patient's reactions).

EAR IRRIGATIONS

Ear irrigations may be done to remove foreign particles from the ear canal such as ceru-

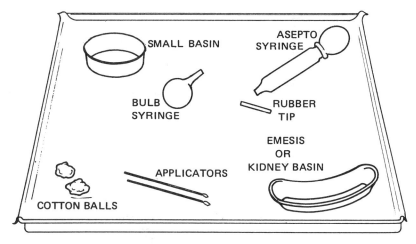

Fig. 17-3 Tray for ear irrigation.

men (wax). They are also used to apply warmth to inflammed and congested ear canals.

The equipment and the procedure is much the same as for an eye irrigation. A tray is prepared containing the following.

- A small, sterile basin containing the solution to be used

- An ear syringe which may be a rubber bulb syringe, an Asepto syringe with a rubber tip, or a sterile metal syringe with a rubber tip

- Sterile cotton balls or gauze sponges
- Sterile cotton-tipped applicators
- A large kidney-shaped basin
- A towel

Procedure

Familiarity with the structures of the ear is necessary before giving an ear irrigation. The patient is told about the procedure, and what will be done.

The medical assistant proceeds in the following way.

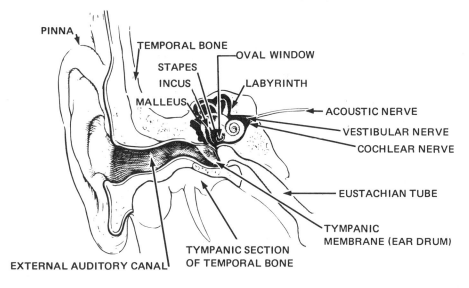

Fig. 17-4 Structures of the ear.

(From Memmler, R. and Rada D. *The Human Body in Health and Disease.* Philadelphia: Lippincott, 1970)

1. Position the patient in a horizontal recumbent position with the head slightly turned toward the affected side (the ear being treated). The towel is placed against the patient's neck to prevent the solution from running down the neck. The emesis or kidney basin is placed directly under the ear to catch the irrigating solution as it runs out of the ear.

2. Remove any visible drainage from the outer canal with the sterile applicators. *Do not probe* into the ear with the applicator. The medical assistant should test the solution for warmth by dropping a small amount of the solution onto her wrist. It should be warm, but not hot. The prescribed temperature for solutions to be used in the ear is 105°-110°F (about 40.6° - 43.3°C). Remember, *the solution is sterile.*

3. Expel the air from the syringe and any solution that might have become cold in the tip of the syringe. Slowly expel the solution from the syringe into the ear canal. The solution should not be forced with a lot of pressure and should be directed to the side of the canal rather than at the eardrum. *Do not block the canal with the syringe.* Room must be allowed for the solution to return past the syringe tip.

4. Continue irrigating until all the prescribed amount of solution is used, or until the returning solution runs clear. If the patient complains of dizziness, nausea, or severe discomfort, discontinue the irrigations and check with the doctor.

5. When all of the solution has been used and the treatment is complete, remove the emesis basin and wipe the patient's neck with a towel. Turn the patient's head so the affected ear will be down toward the treatment table. This will allow

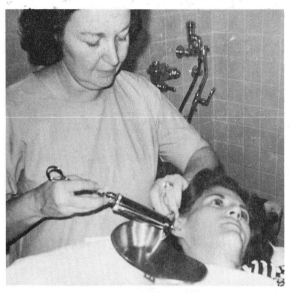

Fig. 17-5 Irrigating the ear.

any excess solution to drain from the ear. Dry the outer ear with the sterile cotton balls or gauze. Do *not* plug the ear with cotton balls or any other packing unless ordered to do so by the physician.

VAGINAL IRRIGATION (DOUCHE)

A vaginal irrigation or douche is given to cleanse the vaginal canal, to remove vaginal secretions, and to apply medication to the vagina. The solution used will depend upon the purpose of the douche. Frequently, one liter (one quart) of solution containing 1 tablespoon of vinegar OR 2 teaspoons of salt is used for cleaning purposes.

The equipment used to give a douche does not have to be sterile unless there has been trauma (damage) to the vaginal tissues. However, the equipment does have to be clean. It must be disinfected or sterilized after every usage.

Today most physician's offices use disposable douche setups that contain all of the necessary equipment. Complete printed instructions on how to use the pack are included. They should be read and thoroughly understood before giving the douche.

It may be necessary to use office equipment and supplies. The following items are necessary for a douche tray.

- A tray with a douche can, rubber tubing and clamp
- A douche nozzle
- Sterile cotton balls and antiseptic solution
- Rubber or disposable gloves
- Forceps
- Towels
- Bedpan
- Douching solution

To prepare the tray for the procedure, remove the douche nozzle from the can and connect it to the end of the rubber tubing; the tubing has a clamp to open and close it off. The other end of the rubber tube is connected to the bottom of the douche can.

The douche solution should be tested carefully for the proper temperature as the vaginal tissues are fairly insensitive to heat. Proper temperature of the solution is 105° - 110°F (40.6° - 43.3°C). The rubber tubing is clamped off before the douche can is filled with the solution.

Procedure

Check with the patient to see if she has ever had a douche before. If not, explain the procedure to the patient as she will need much reassurance during this procedure. The bladder should be emptied before the vaginal irrigation is done. Therefore, the medical assistant may direct the patient to the bathroom.

The medical assistant then proceeds in the following manner.

1. Position the patient in the dorsal recumbent position with the knees bent. The buttocks are placed on the bedpan and the patient made as comfortable as possible. Remember to respect the patient's

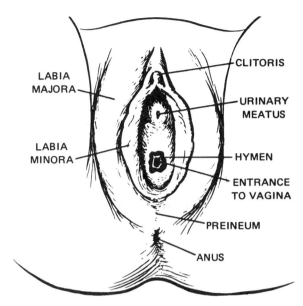

Fig. 17-6 External female genitalia (vulva).

dignity and modesty at all times. Drape her carefully to minimize embarrassment.

2. Put on the rubber or disposable gloves and clean the external area by spreading the labia and wiping downward once with the cotton ball soaked in the antiseptic solution. Repeat until the entire labial area has been cleaned. After each stroke the used cotton ball should be discarded and a new one used for the next stroke. Cotton balls may be discarded into the bedpan (or in a separate basin).

3. After cleaning the labia, allow a *small* amount of the warm douche solution to run over the vulva before inserting the nozzle into the vagina. Be sure the solution is not too warm. The vulva is more sensitive to heat than the vaginal tissues. If the patient feels it is too hot, let the solution cool a bit.

4. Slowly introduce the nozzle into the vagina in a downward and backward direction. Rotate the nozzle carefully, holding the nozzle where the rubber tubing attaches to it. The douche can should be kept approximately 12 to 18 inches

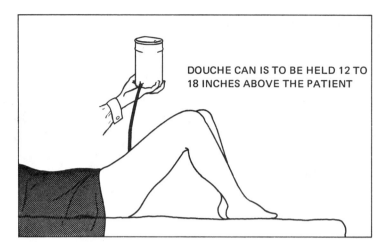

DOUCHE CAN IS TO BE HELD 12 TO 18 INCHES ABOVE THE PATIENT

Fig. 17-7 Height of a douche can.

above the level of the patient's hips to prevent excessive pressure in the vagina.

5. When all solution has been used, clamp the rubber tubing and slowly withdraw the nozzle tip from the vagina. Help the patient into a sitting position on the bedpan to allow all of the douche solution to return.

6. Dry the genital area carefully and remove the bedpan. Have the patient turn on her side and using cotton balls, wipe off any excess water from the posterior area of the vulva and the rectum. Assist the patient from the treatment table and help her to get dressed.

7. Remove all equipment and clean it thoroughly before disinfecting or sterilizing it. Chart the treatment and nature of the returns on the patient's record.

If the patient is to repeat the treatment at home, instruct her to douche, lying in the bathtub with her knees bent. A douche taken while sitting on the toilet is not effective. The flow of gravity prevents the solution from cleansing the entire vaginal area unless the patient is lying down.

ENEMAS

An enema may be considered an irrigation of the lower intestinal tract. Enemas are usu-

ally given to relieve constipation or gas pains. Enemas are also given before x-ray examinations to cleanse the bowel for better visualization. Enemas may be given to instill medication in the rectum.

Procedure

Prepackaged enemas are used in medical offices and are easily administered. Prepackaged enemas are self-contained units with a premeasured amount of solution in a plastic bottle with a lubricated nozzle attached. The plastic bottle is discarded after each use.

The medical assistant proceeds in the following manner.

1. Position the patient on her left side in the Sims' position and drape carefully to avoid embarrassment. The knees should be slightly bent; the bottom leg is extended slightly to help the patient maintain this position. The assistant should be certain that a bedpan is within easy reach as some patients cannot retain solution long enough to get to the bathroom.

2. The buttocks are separated so that the anus can be seen. Check to see that the tip of the enema nozzle is well-lubricated; if not, apply additional lubricant. Gently insert the tip of the nozzle into the rectum. *Do not force the nozzle if resistance*

is present. Gently move the nozzle upward until it is placed about three inches in the rectum.

3. Slowly expel the solution from the bottle into the rectum. When all solution has been emptied, slowly withdraw the nozzle. Discard all equipment that is disposable.

4. If a retention enema was given, allow the patient to rest quietly for a few minutes. If the enema is to be expelled, assist the patient into a sitting position and, then, to the bathroom. Be sure to instruct the patient to take note of the results of the enema or not to flush the toilet so that the assistant can check the results. This is necessary to complete charting of the procedure.

5. Chart the treatment and results of the enema on the patient's record.

SUMMARY

Therapeutic irrigations are administered for several reasons. Eye irrigations are for cleansing and removing foreign particles and to relieve pain and discomfort. Ear irrigations are administered to remove cerumen or other foreign particles and to apply warmth to relieve pain and congestion.

Vaginal irrigations or douches are administered to cleanse the vaginal area or to apply medication to the vagina. Disposable enemas are prepackaged setups that are used to relieve constipation or gas pains, or to instill medication into the rectum.

All treatments are done only upon a physician's order and are carefully charted upon the patient's record. The results of the treatment should accompany the recording of the treatment as well as the time, date, and name of the person administering the treatment.

SUGGESTED ACTIVITIES

• Make arrangements with your instructor to invite an ophthalmologist to speak to the class about eye treatments and irrigations. Discuss the types of solutions that might be used for eye irrigations.

• Practice setting up for eye and ear irrigations.

• Using prepackaged equipment, prepare for administering a douche and enema.

• If there is a practice doll available, administer a douche and an enema. Role play, pretending that the "patient" has never had either treatment before.

REVIEW

Select the answer that best completes the following statements.

1. Solutions that are used for irrigations are

   a. chosen by the medical assistant who administers them.
   b. always prepackaged solutions.
   c. ordered by the physician.
   d. given at room temperature.

2. Syringes used for eye and ear irrigations are always rubber or rubber-tipped because

    a. the syringe must be sterile.
    b. rubber tips prevent possible injury to the patient.
    c. a rubber-tipped syringe is easier to handle.
    d. rubber tips prevent cross-contamination.

3. A small amount of solution is dispelled from the syringe tip before beginning an irrigation because

    a. the solution might have become cold.
    b. the solution might have become contaminated.
    c. the rubber tip might have air bubbles in it.
    d. none of the above.

4. Before beginning the actual irrigation of the ear, the assistant should

    a. probe down to the eardrum to see if the canal is clear.
    b. clean as far down the ear canal as she can with an applicator.
    c. be sure the solution is at least 115°F (46.1°C).
    d. clean the outer ear with an applicator.

5. If the syringe is tightly placed in the ear canal so that the solution cannot return past the syringe,

    a. the eardrum may burst.
    b. the patient might have severe pain.
    c. nausea and vomiting may result.
    d. all of the above.

6. After the irrigation of an ear is complete, the assistant

    a. should dry the ear canal carefully.
    b. turn the head to the opposite side so that the ear can drain.
    c. place cotton balls in the ear to catch excess drainage.
    d. none of the above.

7. The temperature of the solution used for douching must be checked very carefully because

    a. solutions that are too cold are uncomfortable to the patient.
    b. solutions that are too warm are uncomfortable to the patient.
    c. the vaginal tissues are not very sensitive to temperatures.
    d. none of the above.

8. Before giving a vaginal irrigation, the

    a. vulva and labia must be cleaned.
    b. patient must be placed upon a bedpan.
    c. the procedure must be explained to the patient and reassurances given.
    d. all of the above.

9. Enemas may be ordered to

    a. relieve constipation.
    b. relieve gas pains.
    c. instill medications.
    d. all of the above.

10. The assistant must know the results of a cleansing enema in order to

    a. let the patient know the treatment helped him.
    b. be sure she did the treatment correctly.
    c. correctly record the treatment and its results.
    d. none of the above.

11. The height of a douche can

    a. is determined by the height of the bed.
    b. should be no higher than 18 inches above the patient.
    c. is considered of minor importance.
    d. is to be held 8 to 10 inches above the patient.

12. If a retention enema is given,

    a. gently force the nozzle if resistance is present.
    b. it is not necessary to check the results.
    c. allow the patient to rest quietly for a few minutes.
    d. the patient is positioned on her right side.

Unit 18 Physical Therapy

OBJECTIVES

After completing this unit, the student should be able to

- State the purpose of physical therapy.
- State three main classifications of physical therapy.
- Describe the forms of treatment used in each classification.
- Differentiate between a physiatrist and a physical therapist.

There are several methods of treating diseases through the use of physical therapy. The physician who is a specialist in this field is a *physiatrist* and practices physical medicine. A physiatrist has a registered physical therapist to assist with the treatments he or she determines should be given.

Other physicians who order physical therapy for their patients generally send them to a physiatrist or to the nearest hospital that has a physical therapy department. In some states, laws governing medical practice state that no person other than a physician or a registered physical therapist may administer physical therapy. Nevertheless, the medical assistant should be familiar with the various *modalities* (methods) of treatment in order to add to her store of knowledge, and also help the patient.

Physical therapy speeds up the healing processes, relieves pain, improves circulation and motion, and prevents the stiffness of joints and the degeneration of muscles due to lack of use. Physical therapy does not cure disease.

HEAT

Heat may be applied, through physcial therapy, in several ways. Remember, heat increases the circulation of blood and lymph, thereby stimulating weak muscles and facilitating movement as well as relieving pain and stiffness.

Superficial Heat

Superficial or surface heat is a term applied to a method that penetrates the skin to a depth of one to two inches. Surface heat may be applied in several different ways such as heat lamps, hot water bottles, heating pads, *hydroculator packs,* and *infrared radiation.* Hydroculator packs are special packs filled with a heat-retaining substance; they are soaked in very hot water, then wrapped in towels and placed on the patient.

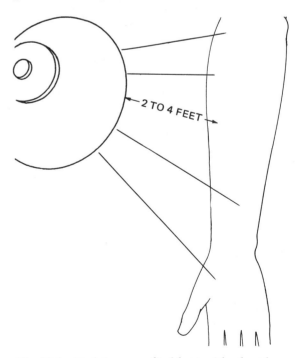

Fig. 18-1 Applying superfical heat with a heat lamp.

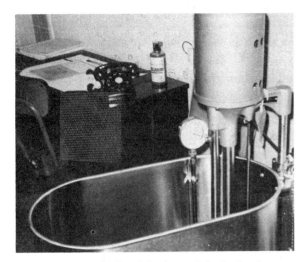

Fig. 18-2 A whirlpool bath used in hydrotherapy.

Before applying *any* heat to a patient, the therapist must be sure that the blood supply to that area is not impaired. If circulation is not adequate, severe burns may result; the impaired circulation will prevent cooling of the heated tissues.

When heat lamps are used, the lamps should be no closer than 2 to 4 feet from the area being treated. If a patient complains of any discomfort from a treatment, the treatment should be discontinued at once.

When *infrared radiation* is used to apply heat, special infrared-producing equipment must be used. This equipment is usually a generator that produces infrared rays in low frequency wavelengths. These infrared wavelengths are called thermal rays, meaning heat rays.

Hydrotherapy

Hydrotherapy, the application of water in the treatment of disease, is a method of physical therapy. Hydrotherapy may consist of soaks, showers, whirlpool baths, or wet packs, using equipment and/or special techniques. Hydrotherapy is administered only by a physician or registered physical therapist. Cold treatments are also included in hydrotherapy.

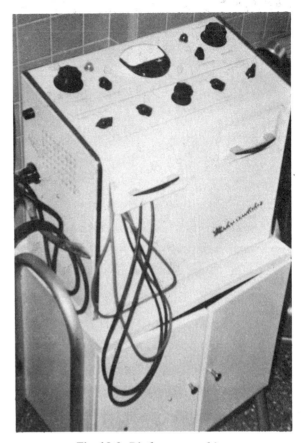

Fig. 18-3 Diathermy machine.

ELECTRICAL CURRENTS

Electrical current may be administered by three methods: *galvanic, sinusoidal,* and *faradic* currents. All three currents are low voltage and are supplied by a special machine for this purpose.

Galvanic current is a direct current that stimulates muscles. It is used when the nerve supply that controls the muscles has been damaged.

Sinusoidal and *faradic currents* are alternating currents, and are useful only if the nerve supply to the muscles is normal. These two currents cause muscle contractions and help the muscles gain strength.

Diathermy

Diathermy is another treatment utilizing electric current. The *diathermy machine* generates short wave currents that create heat in tissues by converting the electrical current or energy into heat. There are many types of diathermy machines. All of them should be operated only by a trained individual since severe burns and injuries may result from improper use of the diathermy apparatus. In the use of diathermy, the patient should barely feel a sensation of heat. At most, only a warm comfortable feeling should be present.

Ultrasonic Therapy

This modality (method) utilizes a special ultrasonic generator that produces vibrations or waves which are faster than sound waves. About a million vibrations or waves are produced each second. The purpose of ultrasonic vibrations is to penetrate very deeply. It can even penetrate bone. Ultrasonic therapy is so effective that it can produce chemical changes deep within tissues. It is used to break up deep scar tissues, relieve deep pain, and in some cases break up calcium deposits that restrict or prevent movement.

MASSAGE

The use of the hands to apply pressure and motion is called massage. It is the oldest kind of physical therapy. Massage is designed to increase circulation, restore motion, relieve pain and tension, and relax muscles. Most persons will benefit from massage; however, it should NOT be used when the following conditions are present.

- Any heart condition, threat of embolism or thrombosis.
- Infections that contain pus.
- Malignant or benign tumors.
- Any wounds that are open such as lacerations or cuts.

There are several kinds of massage used in physical therapy.

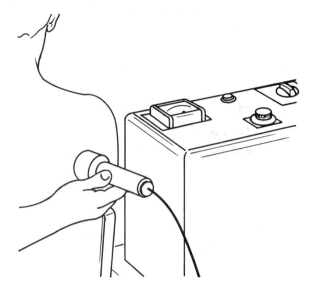

Fig. 18-4 **Application of deep heat, using ultrasonic therapy.**

Effleurage

This is the most frequently-used method of massage. It is easy to use *effleurage.* Gentle pressure is applied to the tissues being massaged. Basically, it is a form of stroking. Backrubs to relieve tension and mild discomfort are an example of effleurage.

Friction

This method of massage is useful in stimulating deeper tissues than are affected by effleurage. Friction massage might be used in deep muscle pain such as cramps in the thigh or calf of the legs.

Petrissage

Petrissage is a rolling and kneading massage. This is very stimulating to structural muscles and results in toning up lax, flaccid (flabby) muscles.

Tapotement

Tapotement is a striking of the body with the hands; it includes clapping with the palms, striking with the side of the hand, punctuating with the tips of the finger, and striking with the clenched hand. It is done with more pressure than the other types of massage and should only be used on a patient by an *experienced therapist.*

Vibration

Vibration is accomplished by using all of the fingertips and gently tapping the body in quick, repeated movements. It produces a very different sensation than does tapotement.

SUMMARY

The purpose of physical therapy is not to cure diseases but to speed up and assist the healing processes, relieve pain, prevent stiffness of joints and muscles, improve circulation and motion, and prevent degeneration of muscle tissue which is due to lack of use.

A physiatrist is a medical specialist who has studied physical medicine. Physical therapy is administered by either the physician or a registered physical therapist.

There are many modalities of physical therapy. Some methods utilize heat, electrical currents, vibrations, water, or massage.

Except for physiatrists and some orthopedic specialists, doctors will not have physical therapy equipment in their office. Patients are usually referred to a hospital with a physical therapy department staffed by registered. qualified personnel. Many states prohibit the practice or administration of physical therapy except by a registered therapist.

SUGGESTED ACTIVITIES

- Make arrangements to visit a local hospital that has a physical therapy department. Arrange for one of the therapists to explain the equipment and how it is used.

- Invite a physical therapist to demonstrate the various types of massage that are used.

REVIEW

A. Answer the following questions.

1. What is the purpose of physical therapy?

2. List the three main classifications of physical therapy.

3. What is a physiatrist?

B.   From column II, select the modality which relates to its description in column I. Fill the blank with the appropriate letter.

Column I	**Column II**

1. _____ The use of thermal or heat rays.   a. hydrotherapy

2. _____ Gentle pressure in a form of stroking.   b. diathermy

3. _____ Shortwave currents that convert the current into heat in the tissues.   c. superficial heat

d. galvanic current

4. _____ Therapy that utilizes water in various ways.   e. ultrasonic therapy

f. faradic current

5. _____ A direct electrical current that stimulates muscles with damaged nerve supplies.   g. effleurage

h. friction

i. petrissage

6. _____ Applied by heat lamps, hot water bottles, and infrared radiation.   j. infrared radiation

k. tapotement

7. _____ Massage that stimulates deep muscles to relieve pain.

8. _____ Alternating current used only when the muscle's nerve supply isn't damaged.

9. _____ A rolling and kneading form of massage.

10. _____ Penetrates into deep muscles and into and through bone.

11. _____ Type of massage which involves striking the body with the hands.

12. _____ Emits a million vibrations per second.

13. _____ Can produce chemical changes deep within the tissues.

14. _____ Penetrates the skin only one to two inches.

15. _____ Produces rays that are low frequency wave lengths.

Unit 19 Catheterization

OBJECTIVES

After completing this unit, the student should be able to

- Distinguish between a French catheter and a Foley or retention catheter.
- Prepare a catheterization tray for the physician.
- Demonstrate how to safely catheterize a female patient.

The medical assistant may not be called upon to catheterize a patient unless she works for a *urologist*. A urologist is a physician who specializes in diseases of the urinary tract. However, there may be occasions when she will be required to do so. Generally, the doctor will catheterize male patients. The assistant may be asked to catheterize female patients. She must be familiar with the structures of the urinary tract before attempting to perform the catheterization, figure 19-1.

PURPOSE

Patients are catheterized to relieve urinary retention, an accumulation of urine which the patient cannot eliminate from the bladder. If a sterile urine specimen is necessary for a required laboratory test, the patient may be catheterized to obtain that urine specimen. Also, if the physician wishes to instill medication into the bladder, the patient's bladder must first be emptied of urine by catheterization.

EQUIPMENT

If disposable catheterization packs are not available, the assistant must prepare the setup. Most offices do use the disposable catheterization packs because they are already packaged sterile and everything needed is pres-

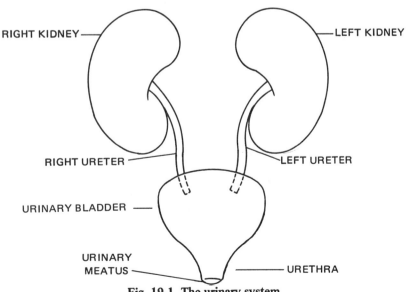

Fig. 19-1 The urinary system.

ent in the pack. However, if a disposable set-up is not available, the following equipment must be assembled:

- A sterile tray covered with a sterile towel
- 2 solution basins (one for the cleansing solution and one to contain the urine received: both sterile)
- Sterile catheters (either French or Foley catheter, size 12 to 16)
- Sterile medicine glass
- Sterile cotton balls
- Sterile 4 x 4 gauze squares
- Specimen bottle with lid (both sterile)
- Sterile forceps
- Sterile drapes for the patient
- Antiseptic solution for cleansing the patient
- Sterile lubricant for the tip of the catheter.

In addition to the equipment on the sterile tray, sterile rubber or disposable gloves will be needed. If the catheter is to remain in the bladder and a Foley catheter is to be used, it will be necessary to inject 5 cc's (5ml) of sterile water to inflate the Foley. Therefore, a sterile syringe, a 25-gauge needle, and a bottle of sterile water for injection will be needed. Good lighting such as that provided by a gooseneck lamp should be available to ensure good visibility during the procedure. The doctor usually inserts an indwelling catheter; however, a medical assistant who has been taught the procedure may be asked to do so.

All of the equipment is assembled on a stand near the treatment table before the procedure is begun.

PROCEDURE

Explain to the patient that you will be inserting a tube in order to remove urine and

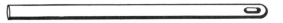

(A) FRENCH CATHETER

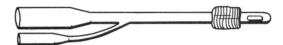

(B) DEFLATED FOLEY CATHETER

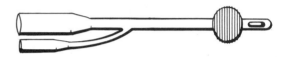

(C) INFLATED FOLEY CATHETER

Fig. 19-2 Urinary catheters.

ask her to relax as much as possible. Cooperation during this procedure will make it easier for the patient and the medical assistant as nervousness on the part of the patient will make the tissues tighten, making it difficult to insert the tube. Also, be sure the bed surface is flat.

1. **Place the patient in a dorsal recumbent position with the knees flexed and ask her to spread her thighs apart. Using a light bath blanket, if available, drape the patient so that only the external genitals will be exposed. Check the gooseneck lamp and adjust it for good visibility.**

2. **Place a sterile towel between the patient's knees and set the sterile setup on this towel. Open the outer wrapping of the sterile setup.**

3. **Wash your hands thoroughly with soap and water. Put on the sterile gloves, pick up the sterile towel and place it between the patient's buttocks and the sterile tray.** *Be very careful not to contaminate the gloved hands.*

4. **Place the cotton balls in the antiseptic solution. Place a small amount of the lubricant on a 4 x 4 inch gauze square. Remove the catheter from its protective wrapping and place it in the empty basin. Remove the lid from the specimen container. Remember:** *all articles are sterile and must remain on the sterile field.*

5. **Separate the labia with the fingers of the gloved** *left* **hand. It will remain in this position until the procedure is completed.** *Since this hand has touched the patient*

it has become contaminated and must not touch the sterile field again. With the right hand, touch the tip of the catheter to the lubricant on the 4 x 4 inch gauze square, being careful not to obstruct the opening at the tip of the catheter. Lay the catheter aside (temporarily) with the tip lying on a sterile 4 x 4 inch gauze square.

6. Using the forceps with the right hand, pick up a cotton ball soaked with the antiseptic solution and wipe down the middle of the labia and *discard* the cotton ball. Then wipe down one side of the labia and discard the cotton ball. Repeat with the other side of the labia. Follow the same procedure until the entire area has been cleansed. After each stroke with the cotton ball, it is discarded into a nonsterile container. This may be an emesis basin or paper bag outside of the sterile field. The cotton ball must not be placed back on the sterile field.

7. After cleaning the area, locate the urinary meatus. Use only the left hand to hold the labia open. Do not touch the patient with the right hand as it must be used only to handle sterile objects. The meatus is located *below the clitoris* and *above the vaginal opening.* It should not be difficult to locate unless there is edema or other abnormalities.

8. Pick up the lubricated catheter with the thumb and index finger of the right hand about 3 to 4 inches from the tip. Be sure the basin is ready for the urine. It may be wise to rest the end of the catheter in the basin, keeping the basin close to the patient so the catheter may be inserted freely. Gently insert the tip about 2 to 3 inches into the urethra. The flow of urine should begin immediately.

    CAUTION: If the catheter becomes contaminated, use another. Do not force the catheter if there is any resistance. Do *not insert the catheter any further than 3 inches* as it may rupture the bladder wall.

9. Let the first flow of urine run into the basin used to collect the urine. Then close the catheter off with the right gloved, sterile hand and place the open end into the sterile specimen bottle. When a sufficient amount of urine has been obtained for the specimen, the flow of urine may be directed back into the basin used for collection. When the flow of urine stops, gently withdraw the catheter. Dry the area with the remaining cotton balls. Put the lid on the specimen container and remove the tray from the table. Make the patient comfortable.

10. Measure the total amount of urine, both in the specimen container and in the basin. (This is to be recorded on the patient's records.) Label the specimen con-

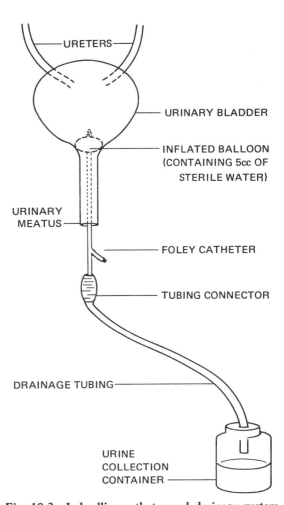

Fig. 19-3 Indwelling catheter and drainage system.

tainer immediately. Include the patient's name, the date, and the name of the doctor. Clean and sterilize all equipment. If a disposable pack has been used, all of its contents are discarded. Record the entire procedure and the results on the patient's record. This includes the character of the return flow such as the presence of cloudiness, particles, mucus, etc.

When a catheterization is performed to place an indwelling catheter in the bladder, the procedure is the same except that *after* the catheter is in place in the bladder *and the bladder has been emptied,* 5 milliliters (5 cc's) of sterile water in the syringe is injected into the small rubber membrane that forks off the catheter near the open end. This inflates a small balloon type structure near the tip of the catheter that prevents the catheter from slipping out of the bladder, figure 19-3.

SUMMARY

Catheterizations are performed to relieve retention, obtain a sterile urine specimen, or to instill medication after the bladder has been emptied. They are performed only when the medical assistant has demonstrated ability to perform the procedure and is authorized by the doctor.

The entire procedure must be performed very carefully in order to maintain sterile conditions throughout the procedure. Any break in technique requires that the procedure be repeated. Poor or careless aseptic technique can result in a very severe bladder infection and/or cystitis (inflammation of the urinary tract).

A French catheter is used for simple catheterizations and a Foley or indwelling catheter is used if the catheter is to remain in the bladder.

SUGGESTED ACTIVITIES

- Without referring to the text, prepare a setup for a catheterization. Check the items against the list in the unit.

- Practice catheterization on a practice doll if one is available. Demonstrate the procedure for your instructor's evaluation.

- Research the term "cystitis" to find the causes, signs, and symptoms.

- Discuss some of the possible dangers of catheterizations.

REVIEW

Select the answer that best completes the following statements.

1. The antiseptic solution found on a catheterization tray is used to
   a. lubricate the catheter before insertion.
   b. instill into the bulb that holds the Foley catheter in place.
   c. clean the external genitals before catheterization.
   d. none of the above.

2. The passage through which the catheter passes to reach the bladder is called the
   a. ureter   c. meatus
   b. labia   d. urethra

3. The forceps contained in the catheterization setup are used to
   a. pinch off the catheter.
   b. hold the cotton balls used to clean the labia.
   c. spread the labia so the meatus can be seen.
   d. hold the 4 x 4 inch gauze squares.

4. A catheter that is put in the bladder and allowed to remain after the procedure is complete is called a(n)
   a. indwelling catheter.
   b. retention catheter.
   c. Foley catheter.
   d. all of the above.

5. A catheter might be allowed to remain in the bladder because

    a. the patient cannot void.
    b. urinary retention is present.
    c. loss of bladder control exists.
    d. all of the above.

6. For catheterization purposes, the catheter is inserted

    a. from 2 to 3 inches.
    b. about one inch.
    c. from 3 to 4 inches.
    d. none of the above.

Unit 20 Collection of Specimens

OBJECTIVES

After completing this unit, the student should be able to

- State the principles for collecting specimens.
- Explain how to collect specimens of urine, feces, sputum, and blood.
- Cite precautions to be taken in the collection of specimens.

The general principles for collecting specimens are the same for all types of specimens. If the assistant learns and applies these basic principles, the collection of any specimen will not be difficult even if someone else does the collecting.

The patient must fully understand *what* is to be collected, *how* it is to be collected, and *what* container will be used.

Proper storage of the specimen is necessary until it reaches the laboratory. If the patient is collecting the specimen he must be given the proper collecting container. In some cases, a preservative must be added to the container to preserve the specimen until the tests can be run.

Proper labeling of the specimen container is vital. Label the container before giving it to the patient. If the specimen is collected in the office, it must be labeled with the patient's full name, the doctor's name and the date. A laboratory request accompanies the specimen if it is sent to an outside laboratory; if the patient takes the specimen (for example, from his home) the medical assistant must call the laboratory beforehand and indicate what tests the doctor has ordered.

URINE SPECIMENS

The patient is given a disposable urine collection cup or container with a lid and asked to urinate into it. The assistant must be certain that the patient understands what is to be collected. The patient is taken to the bathroom and asked to please return the specimen after it has been collected. Promptly label the specimen and take it to the laboratory with a request slip stating the tests to be made. If a routine urinalysis is to be done, the container should be clean but does not need to be sterile.

If the urine specimen is to be a "clean-catch" specimen, this means the patient must be very careful not to contaminate the specimen while collecting it. The patient is instructed to clean the external genitals (penis of male or vulva of female) before voiding into the container. Prepackaged, moistened gauze sponges which contain a skin antiseptic are used for this purpose. Care must be taken not to allow the pubic hair to touch the container.

If the urine specimen is a "midstream" specimen, the patient is instructed to clean the external genitals thoroughly, pass a small amount of urine, and then direct the urine from

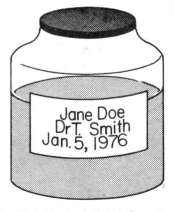

Fig. 20-1 Correctly labeled specimen.

the midstream flow into the sterile container. This action of voiding a small amount first, avoids the possibility of microorganisms around the external urinary meatus from entering the urine specimen. Both clean-catch and midstream specimens are labeled as such.

FECAL SPECIMENS

Specimens of feces are normally collected at home by the patient. The patient is given a labeled, disposable collection cup which also has a cap, and several tongue depressors. He is instructed to have his next bowel movement in some container from which he can obtain the necessary stool specimen. The feces (stool) is then transferred from the container to the specimen cup with the tongue blades. The tongue blades are then discarded.

Some specimens must be preserved in solution until they reach the laboratory. The patient must be given the preservative if this is the case. Other tests which may be ordered require that the feces be examined promptly; that is, as close to body temperature as possible. If this is necessary inform the patient so that proper arrangements can be made.

SPUTUM SPECIMENS

Sputum specimens must be collected in the early morning as soon as the patient arises. Instructions are given in the doctor's office, and the patient is given a sterile, disposable container with a cap. The assistant must be absolutely certain that the patient understands that sputum is mucus coughed up from the lungs and *not* saliva from the mouth. This is the most frequent reason for improper collection of sputum specimens. Explain to the patient that he must not allow anything but sputum to touch the inside of the specimen container. After the sputum has been collected, the container is tightly capped and taken to the laboratory. The laboratory must be notified of the

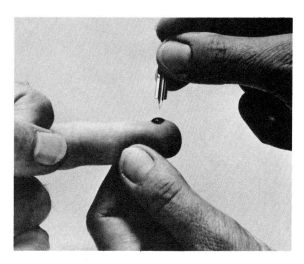

Fig 20-2 Use of a lancet.

tests to be made. Remember that the container must be labeled. Labeling may be done *before* giving the container to the patient.

BLOOD SPECIMENS

Blood may be collected in two ways in the doctor's office, from the finger and from the vein. For testing small amounts of blood, the skin is punctured. This procedure is sometimes called a "finger stick." In an adult, the finger is used as the puncture sight. In infants, the heel or the big toe is used. CAUTION: Never take a blood sample from any area that is edematous, scarred, calloused, or bruised.

A lancet is used to puncture the skin, figure 20-2. Choose the sight and gently squeeze from the base toward the tip. Cleanse the area carefully with an alcohol sponge. (Prepackaged or cotton balls soaked in isopropyl alcohol may be used). Allow the finger to dry without touching the cleansed area. Grasp the finger firmly at the middle or first joint and hold it securely to prevent jerking when the lancet punctures the skin. Holding the blood lancet firmly in the right hand, quickly insert it 3 to 4 millimeters into the surface of the palm side of the finger. This must be done with a quick, stabbing motion. It is no more painful to make a 3 millimeter puncture than a 1

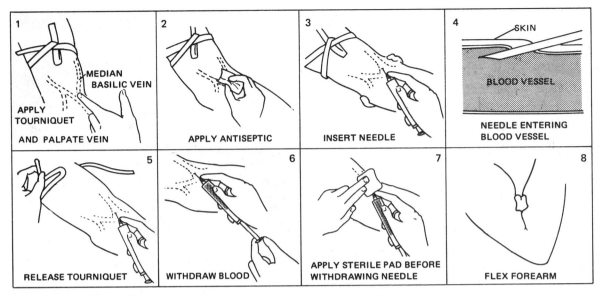

Fig. 20-3 How to collect a venous blood specimen.

millimeter puncture that might have to be repeated. When done correctly, there is an immediate flow of blood.

Wipe the first drops of blood off the finger with a dry sterile cotton sponge. Do not squeeze the finger as this will dilute the blood with cellular fluid.

Gentle pressure will speed the next drop of blood which can be obtained with a pipette for the blood count.

A single puncture effectively done, can provide enough blood for a complete blood count. However, as a new drop of blood should be used for each count, several pipettes of blood must be obtained from the same puncture.

If a larger quantity of blood is needed for testing, a *venipuncture* is done. This is the insertion of a needle into a vein (usually the median basilic vein) in order to withdraw several milliliters of blood. Special vacuum tubes equipped with needles are available. Otherwise the medical assistant may use a sterile syringe with a 1 to 1½ inch, 20-gauge sterile needle. Before attempting the venipuncture, a tourniquet and alcohol sponges (70% isopropyl alcohol) should also be ready for use. *The*

medical assistant must have the permission of the doctor and adequate training to perform the procedure.

Remember, you are introducing a foreign object directly into the bloodstream so your technique must be aseptically flawless.

The patient is seated in a comfortable position and the assistant explains what is to be done. The inner aspect of the arm at the elbow, is inspected to see if the vein will be suitable for venipuncture. As stated previously, the assistant never takes a blood sample from a scarred, bruised or edematous area. Also, avoid using a vein which appears engorged (full of "knots").

Apply the tourniquet above the elbow. Ask the patient to open and close his hand. When the site of injection has been determined, cleanse the area carefully with an alcohol sponge. Let the skin dry completely. If a sterile syringe and needle are being used, be sure there is no air in the syringe.

Placing the left hand behind the patient's elbow, draw the skin (with the fingers and thumb) toward the back of the elbow. Visually locate the vein and with a sure quick movement, insert the needle upward into the vein. Aspirate to be certain the needle is securely in the vein. If blood returns in the syringe rapidly, hold the needle steady and release the tourniquet with the left hand. Draw as much blood as needed into the syringe (the size of the syringe is determined by the amount of blood required). Holding a clean alcohol sponge in the left hand, remove the needle from the vein. Immediately place the alcohol sponge over the puncture. Ask the patient to apply pressure over the sponge for several minutes and to flex the forearm, figure 20-3. If this is not done, the vein will bleed under the skin and result in a blue bruise.

While the patient holds the sponge over the puncture, detach the needle and empty the contents of the syringe into a test tube which contains an anticoagulent that prevents clotting. After this anticoagulent is added, the specimen becomes *oxalated blood.* The test tube is tightly stoppered and shaken for three minutes. The tube must be labeled immediately with the patient's name, the doctor's name, and the date. The needle and syringe must be soaked in a blood-dissolving solution unless a disposable set is used.

SUMMARY

To collect specimens for laboratory studies, the patient's cooperation is absolutely nec-

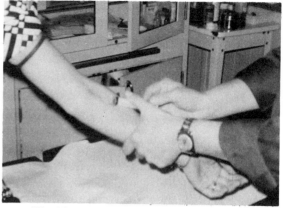

Fig. 20-4 Withdrawing a venous specimen.

essary. The correct specimen must be collected in the correct container and in the correct manner in order to have a specimen that can be properly tested.

All specimens are labeled with the patient's first and last name, the doctor's name, and the date. If the tests are to be made in a laboratory other than the doctor's office, a request must be sent to the laboratory. The doctor receives the results.

Specimens must be preserved or stored in the proper manner until the laboratory can test them. The assistant must be familiar with the different types of tests in order to know whether a preservative is necessary or not. Some assistants maintain a small file box with an index card containing the specifics for each laboratory test.

SUGGESTED ACTIVITIES

- Observe a laboratory technician doing finger sticks and venipunctures.

- Practice instructing each other to collect various types of specimens such as urine, feces, and sputum.

- Practice finger stick punctures on each other, pipetting the blood, and explaining the procedure as if the classmate were a patient.

- Practice venipuncture technique on a practice "arm" model if one is available. If one is not available, practice on a classmate under the strict supervision of your instructor. Remember, you are introducing a foreign object directly into the bloodstream so your technique must be aseptically flawless.

REVIEW

Select the answer that best completes the following statements.

1. The patient may collect the following specimens at home

   a. feces.
   b. urine.
   c. sputum.
   d. all of these.

2. One of the most frequent reasons why sputum specimens are improperly collected is

   a. the specimen is collected in the wrong type container.
   b. the patient forgets to collect the specimen at the right time.
   c. the proper preservative is not used.
   d. the patient doesn't understand what sputum is and collects saliva instead.

3. To do a finger puncture correctly, the assistant must

   a. clean the finger tip properly.
   b. puncture the finger 3 to 4 mm deep.
   c. wipe off the first drop of blood.
   d. all of the above.

4. A "clean-catch" specimen is one that is

   a. simply caught in a specimen cup or container.
   b. collected in midstream flow.
   c. collected after the external genitals have been thoroughly cleaned.
   d. none of the above.

5. Specimens of feces are usually collected

   a. at home.
   b. at the doctor's office.
   c. at the laboratory.
   d. at all of the these places.

6. Oxalated blood is blood that has been

   a. collected by venipuncture.
   b. stored for later use.
   c. preserved by adding anticoagulants.
   d. obtained by finger puncture.

7. Tightly squeezing the finger after a small puncture will result in

   a. a heavier flow of blood.
   b. diluted blood.
   c. severe pain.
   d. all of these.

8. Sterile precautions need NOT be followed in the collection of the following specimen

   a. venipuncture.
   b. finger puncture.
   c. sputum collection.
   d. routine urinalysis.

9. Do not attempt to obtain blood from any area that is

   a. scarred.
   b. calloused.
   c. bruised.
   d. all of these.

Self-Evaluation Test 3

Select the answers that best complete the following statements.

1. A skin prep is done to prepare a surgical site for an incision by removing

   a. dirt.
   b. hair.
   c. germs.
   d. all of these.

2. Postoperative instructions are given to the patient

   a. by the physician.
   b. by the medical assistant.
   c. by the receptionist.
   d. by mail.

3. In any treatment administered to the patient in the doctor's office, the responsibilities of the medical assistant are

   a. to prepare the patient.
   b. to prepare the treatment room.
   c. to assist the physician.
   d. all of the above.

4. A surgical drape is a supply that is used exclusively

   a. to prepare the treatment room.
   b. after surgery to protect the wound.
   c. during the surgical procedure.
   d. preoperatively.

5. A covering that is used to protect an open wound is a

   a. dressing.
   b. bandage.
   c. cast.
   d. plaster of paris.

6. Usually triangular bandages are used as

   a. dressing to hold a bandage securely.
   b. bandages applied to movable parts of the body.
   c. pressure bandages to prevent hemorrhage.
   d. supports to injured extremities.

7. When heat is applied to a part of the body, the results are

   a. an excess of blood accumulating in that part.
   b. relaxation of muscles, tendons, and ligaments.
   c. both of the above.
   d. neither of the above.

8. Moist heat is generally applied by using

   a. a heating pad.
   b. a heat light.
   c. warm compresses.
   d. all of these.

9. The solution being used to soak compresses should not be in excess of
   a. 212°F (100°C).   c. 125°F (51.7°C).
   b. 115°F (46.1°C).   d. none of these.

10. If cold compresses are left for too long a time on a patient, the results will be
   a. injury to the circulatory system.
   b. freezing of the area being treated.
   c. infection due to lowered resistance.
   d. the same as if the compresses were hot.

11. The abbreviation used for both eyes is
   a. O.D.   c. O.S.
   b. A.U.   d. O.U.

12. Ear irrigations are given for several reasons. Which of the following reasons is not a valid one
   a. to remove cerumen.
   b. to apply heat.
   c. to remove a small dried object.
   d. to apply medication to the ear.

13. A douche must be sterile and given under sterile technique when
   a. there has been trauma such as a break in the membrane.
   b. the patient has an infectious discharge.
   c. after the patient has given birth to a child.
   d. the patient is a young girl.

14. When administering a douche to a patient, she is placed in the
   a. lateral position with the knees flexed.
   b. sitting position on the toilet or commode.
   c. dorsal recumbent position with the knees bent.
   d. jackknife position.

15. The choice of electrical current that would be used in physical therapy in a case where the nerves that control the muscles have been damaged would be
   a. diathermy.   c. sinusoidal current.
   b. galvanic current.   d. faradic current.

16. The type of physical therapy that would be used to break up scar tissue would be
   a. diathermy.   c. ultrasonic therapy.
   b. hydrotherapy.   d. effleurage.

17. The catheter with a small balloon on the tip which is inserted into the bladder and inflated to hold the catheter in place is called a
   a. French catheter.   c. nasal catheter.
   b. Foley catheter.   d. urethral catheter.

18. For withdrawing urine, the catheter should be inserted into the meatus for a distance of about

    a. 3 to 4 inches.   c. 5 inches.
    b. 2 to 3 inches.   d. one-half inch.

19. A lubricant is used during insertion of the catheter to

    a. prevent pain and discomfort.
    b. avoid tissue damage.
    c. make insertion of the catheter easier.
    d. do all of the above.

20. If the tip of the catheter touches the patient's thigh during the catheterization, the assistant

    a. continues with the catheterization procedure.
    b. may wipe the catheter with a sterile sponge and then continue.
    c. replaces it with another sterile catheter.
    d. dips the catheter into the lubricant.

Section 4
Administration of Medications

Unit 21 Terms Used in Drug Administration

OBJECTIVES

After studying this unit, the student should be able to

- Differentiate between the terms, pharmacology and chemotherapy.
- State three sources of drug information.
- Write abbreviations, signs and symbols used in the administration of medications.
- Convert Roman numerals and Arabic numbers.

There are many terms, abbreviations, signs, and symbols used in the administration of medications that the medical assistant must know and use.

Drugs are substances that are used as medicines. They may be administered in various ways and strengths.

The treatment of disease is called *therapy*. *Therapeutic* refers to methods of therapy.

Chemotherapy is the treatment of disease by the use of drugs (chemical substances) that act on the microorganism causing the disease. Diseases are also treated with other chemical agents in addition to drugs.

Pharmacology is the study of drugs and their actions. Anyone administering medications must have some knowledge of pharmacology. There are many sources of information about the study of drugs and how they affect the body systems. A few are described here:

- *The Pharmacopoeia of the United States of America* (USP) and *The National Formulary* (NF). Drugs listed in these books are official drugs that conform to national drug standards. Detailed information is given relating to the usefulness, toxicity, source, chemistry, dosage, and other points of drugs. Both the National Formulary and The Pharmacopoeia of the United States of America are legal standard books for drugs.

- *Pharmacopoeia Internationalis.* This is an international drug book that strives to standardize drugs worldwide.

- *The Physicians' Desk Reference* (PDR). This book includes the latest information obtained from drug manufacturers about their products. It is found in many offices and must be kept current. Supplements are periodically issued and changes must be noted in the doctor's copy.

ABBREVIATIONS

There are many abbreviations used in the prescribing and administration of medications, figure 21-1. The assistant must memorize these and be prepared to use them correctly.

In addition to the abbreviations given in figure 21-1, there are other signs and symbols the assistant must learn.

Abbreviations	Meaning	Abbreviations	Meaning
a̅a̅	of each	NPO	nothing by mouth
a.c.	before meals	O	pint
ad lib	as desired	o.d.	right eye
aq.	water	o.s.	left eye
b.i.d.	twice a day	oz.	ounce
c̅	with	p.c.	after meals
caps.	capsule	p.o.	by mouth
cc	cubic centimeter	PRN	as required or as necessary
Disc.	discontinue	q.d.	every day
dil.	dilute	q.h.	every hour
dr.	dram	q. 2h.	every 2 hours
elix.	elixer	q. 4h.	every 4 hours
ext.	extract	q.i.d.	four times a day
gal.	gallon	q.o.d.	every other day
Gm	gram	q.s.	sufficient quantity
gr.	grain	s̅	without
gtt.	drop	sp.	spirits
gtts.	drops	s̅s̅	half
(H)	per hypodermic	stat.	immediately
h.	hour	sub cu	subcutaneous (under the skin)
H.S.	hour of sleep	(SC, Subc	
I.M.	intramuscular	or s.c.)	
I.V.	intravenous	syr.	syrup
ℳ	minum	tab.	tablet
mg	milligram	t.i.d.	three times a day
ml	milliliter	tr. or tinct.	tincture
noc.	at night	ung.	ointment

Fig. 21-1 Abbreviations used in drug administration.

Roman	Arabic	Roman	Arabic
I	1	XVIII	18
II	2	XIX	19
III	3	XX	20
IV	4	XXI	21
V	5	XXII	22
VI	6	XXIII	23
VII	7	XXIV	24
VIII	8	XXV	25
IX	9	XXVI	26
X	10	XXVII	27
XI	11	XXVIII	28
XII	12	XXIX	29
XIII	13	XXX	30
XIV	14	XL	40
XV	15	L	50
XVI	16	C	100
XVII	17	M	1000

Fig. 21-2 Roman and Arabic numbers.

Sign, Symbol	Meaning
@	at
ʒ	dram
℥	ounce
O	pint
C	gallon

The symbols for amounts listed above are used with Roman Numerals. Example:

1. ʒ̄ī   means two drams
2. ℥ss   means one-half ounce
3. ʒīss   means one and one-half drams

Obviously, this means that the student must know the Roman numerals as well as the Arabic numbers, figure 21-2, page 125.

SUMMARY

The medical office assistant must learn *terminology* (the study of words) relating to pharmacology and the administration of drugs. In addition, the assistant must know the abbreviations, signs, symbols, and method of use for these terms. Also necessary is a working knowledge of Roman numerals and the sources of drug information which are official and conform to national legal standards.

SUGGESTED ACTIVITIES

- Practice writing the abbreviations, signs, and symbols used in this unit.
- Study one or more of the recommended sources for drug information and list the general contents. Share information with your classmates.

REVIEW

A. Define pharmacology and chemotherapy.

B. Write the abbreviation, sign, or symbol for the following terms.

1. after meals   _____
2. tablet   _____
3. every 4 hours   _____
4. hour of sleep   _____
5. milligram   _____
6. left eye   _____
7. as necessary   _____
8. gram   _____
9. cubic centimeter   _____
10. subcutaneous   _____
11. three times a day   _____
12. grain   _____
13. by mouth   _____
14. ounce   _____

15. ointment   _____

16. nothing by mouth   _____

17. dram   _____

18. every other day   _____

19. gallon   _____

20. minum   _____

21. milliliter   _____

22. pint   _____

23. drop   _____

24. sufficient quantity   _____

25. immediately   _____

C. Fill the blank with the correct Roman numerals

  1. 4   _____

  2. 32   _____

  3. 7   _____

  4. 51   _____

  5. 100   _____

  6. 24   _____

  7. 45   _____

  8. 58   _____

  9. 12   _____

10. 90   _____

11. 1001   _____

12. 89   _____

13. 10   _____

14. 19   _____

D. Fill the blank with the correct Arabic numbers.

  1. XV _____   6. XXIX _____

  2. C _____   7. VI _____

  3. IX _____   8. XIV _____

  4. CC _____   9. M _____

  5. LIX _____   10. XL _____

E.   In longhand, write out the instruction written below.

1. *Tabs ii q.i.d., p.o.*

2. *Give 0.5 Gm p.o., b.i.d.*

3. *℥ iv p.o., q. 4 h.*

4. *Give 50 mg I.M., q.d.*

5. *℥ viii p.o., q.o.d.*

6. *Caps ii @ h.s., p.o.*

7. *Give 2 cc Subc., t.i.d.*

Unit 22 Mathematics Review

OBJECTIVES

After studying this unit, the student should determine weaknesses and be able to

- Add, subtract, multiply, and divide fractions.
- Add, subtract, multiply, and divide decimals and whole numbers.
- Convert fractions, decimals and percentages.
- Change ratios to percents, fractions or decimals.
- Find the unknown quantity in ratio-proportion problems.

The medical assistant may be called upon to administer medications to patients. SHE DOES THIS ONLY BY PERMISSION OF THE PHYSICIAN AND UNDER HIS SUPERVISION. No medical assistant should assume she has the authority to prepare drugs for use or administer them to patients. The physician is responsible for the patient's safety and may delegate duties to his medical assistant.

In order to compute dosage and convert from one system of measurement to another, the medical assistant must have a working knowledge of mathematics; this includes knowing the metric and the apothecaries' system of weights and measurements. This unit consists of a review of basic mathematics.

FRACTIONS AND MIXED NUMBERS

1. Express these fractions in their lowest terms.

   a. $\frac{18}{36}$ = _____   e. $\frac{150}{200}$ = _____

   b. $\frac{4}{16}$ = _____   f. $\frac{16}{72}$ = _____

   c. $\frac{150}{175}$ = _____   g. $\frac{9}{81}$ = _____

   d. $\frac{5}{100}$ = _____   h. $\frac{75}{300}$ = _____

   i. $\frac{12}{144}$ = _____   j. $\frac{6}{120}$ = _____

2. Change these fractions to mixed numbers.

   a. $\frac{75}{25}$ = _____   f. $\frac{15}{4}$ = _____

   b. $\frac{16}{4}$ = _____   g. $\frac{56}{7}$ = _____

   c. $\frac{11}{5}$ = _____   h. $\frac{34}{17}$ = _____

   d. $\frac{144}{10}$ = _____   i. $\frac{21}{9}$ = _____

   e. $\frac{99}{3}$ = _____   j. $\frac{13}{2}$ = _____

3. Change these mixed numbers to fractions.

   a. $2\frac{4}{5}$ = _____   f. $17\frac{2}{3}$ = _____

   b. $50\frac{2}{3}$ = _____   g. $11\frac{1}{8}$ = _____

   c. $4\frac{3}{4}$ = _____   h. $28\frac{9}{10}$ = _____

   d. $3\frac{7}{8}$ = _____   i. $6\frac{3}{4}$ = _____

   e. $2\frac{5}{7}$ = _____   j. $31\frac{2}{11}$ = _____

4. Add the following fractions. Use the space to show calculations. Enter the

answer on the line. Reduce answers to lowest terms.

a. 14 1/4 + 16 3/4 + 20 1/2   = _____

b. 10 1/8 + 22 3/4 + 17 2/3   = _____

c. 1 1/6 + 21 1/4 + 34 1/3   = _____

d. 99 3/8 + 4 3/4 + 15 1/6   = _____

e. 25 5/8 + 11 3/4 + 9/10   = _____

5. Subtract the following fractions. Show calculations. Reduce answers to lowest terms.

a. 9/10 – 3/5   = _____

b. 8/16 – 2/8   = _____

c. 7/8 – 3/16   = _____

d. 2 3/4 – 1 1/2   = _____

e. 125 3/25 – 75 2/50   = _____

6. Multiply the following fractions. Show calculations. Reduce answers to lowest terms.

a. 4/5 x 1/4   = _____

b. 1 1/2 x 6 5/8   = _____

c. 2/5 x 1/6 x 3/4   = _____

d. 6 3/4 x 10 2/9   = _____

e. 2/3 x 3/4 x 4/5   = _____

7. Divide the following fractions and reduce answers to lowest terms.

a. 3/8 ÷ 5/6   = _____

b. 4/6 ÷ 6/12   = _____

c. 1/150 ÷ 1/200   = _____

d. 50 ÷ 12 1/2   = _____

e. 22 1/2 ÷ 3 1/8   = _____

DECIMALS

1. Change the following decimals to fractions. Reduce to lowest terms.
   a. 0.50   = _____

   b. 1.75   = _____

   c. 3.40   = _____

   d. .005   = _____

   e. 10.2   = _____

2. Change the following fractions to decimals.
   a. 2/5   = _____

   b. 1/100 = _____

   c. 3/4   = _____

   d. 7/10   = _____

e. 3/8   = _____

3. Add the following decimals. Show calculations.
   a. 0.65, 1.247, 9.99   = _____

   b. 28, 0.0045, 0.10   = _____

   c. 1, 101, .0011, 0.1   = _____

   d. 45.67, 22.009, 0.003 = _____

   e. 7.42, 8.006, 9.0810   = _____

4. Subtract the following decimals.
   a. 75.67 – 62.008   = _____

   b. 4.1 – 3.9   = _____

   c. 999.9 – .9999   = _____

d. 22 – 3.6   = _____

b. 0.006 ÷ 0.050   = _____

e. 700 – 86.0001   = _____

c. 250 ÷ 0.25   = _____

5. Multiply the following decimals.

a. 7 x 9.15   = _____

d. 8 ÷ 0.005   = _____

e. 9.72 ÷ 2.700   = _____

b. 7.5 x 3.117   = _____

PERCENTAGES

1. Change the following fractions and decimals to percent.

c. 1.234 x 100.07   = _____

a. 0.14	= _____	f. 17/20	= _____
b. .275	= _____	g. 1/25	= _____
c. .075	= _____	h. 3/50	= _____
d. 9.02	= _____	i. 3/1000	= _____
e. .001	= _____	j. 1/3	= _____

d. 0.0003 x 0.002   = _____

RATIOS AND PROPORTIONS

1. Show the following fractions, decimals, and percents as ratios.

e. 150 x 0.5   = _____

a. 4/15   = _____

6. Divide the following decimals.

b. 3/8   = _____

a. 100 ÷ 2.5   = _____

c. 38/99 = _____

d. 1%   = _____

e. 0.8%   = _____

2. Find the unknown quantity, X, in the following proportions. Show calculations. Enter answers on line.

   a. 5:400 :: X:80   = _____

   b. 1/4:1 :: 1/6:X   = _____

   c. X:40 :: 3:12   = _____

   d. 0.06:X :: 0.25:20   = _____

e. 30:80 :: X:64   = _____

If any difficulty is encountered in working these mathematic problems, study basic mathematics until these problems can be solved with ease.

SUMMARY

The medical assistant may be allowed to administer medications *if the physician delegates this responsibility to her.* Therefore, she must have a workable knowledge of mathematics. A knowledge of mathematics is essential in order to compute dosage and to convert dosage from one system to another. Computation of dosage is necessary in giving medications. Medications are *never* administered without the supervision and permission of the physician.

SUGGESTED ACTIVITIES

- Using a math workbook or textbook recommended by the instructor, or using problems prepared by the instructor, practice the following math exercises:

   Fractions: addition, subtraction, multiplication, division.
   Decimals: addition, subtraction, multiplication, division.
   Percentages: fractions and decimals.
   Ratio: fractions, decimals, and whole numbers.
   Proportions: solving for X, with fractions, decimals, and whole numbers.

Unit 23 Systems of Measurement

OBJECTIVES

After studying this unit, the student should be able to

- Identify the prefixes of the metric system.
- Recite the units of volume and weight given in the metric system.
- Recite the units of volume and weight given in the apothecaries' system.
- Convert dosages from the apothecaries' system to the metric system.

THE METRIC SYSTEM

The metric system of measurement is based upon the decimal system where division and multiples of a unit are in ratios of ten. This is the most accurate and flexible system. to use and is easy to work with because the basic unit is the liter, the gram or the meter. The medical assistant will be working with liters and grams and their prefixes. (Other terms belong to other systems of measurement).

- The metric units.

  liter (L) . . . . fluid volume
  gram (Gm) . . . . . solid weight
  meter (m) . . . . . distance

- The prefixes that indicate divisions of metric units.

  deci . . . . 0.1 of the unit
  centi . . . . . 0.01 of the unit
  milli . . . . . . 0.001 of the unit

- The prefixes that indicate multiples of metric units.

  deka . . . . 10 times the unit
  hecto . . . . 100 times the unit
  kilo . . . . . 1000 times the unit

The medical assistant should be familiar with the tables of metric volume and weight, and also be able to recognize differences between prefixes, figure 23-1.

The units of volume and weight shown in figure 23-2 must be memorized by anyone who expects to compute dosage of medication and administer medicines.

Arabic numbers and decimal fractions are used in the metric system. No period follows the abbreviation and the numbers are always written before the abbreviation (for example, 5 mg). This differs from the apothecaries' system where the numbers should follow the symbol or abbreviation (℥ⁱⁱ and gr v). Although Roman numerals are most frequently

VOLUME				WEIGHT			
0.1	liter	= 1	deciliter	0.1	gram	= 1	decigram
0.01	liter	= 1	centimeter	0.01	gram	= 1	centigram
0.001	liter	= 1	milliliter	0.001	gram	= 1	milligram
10.0	liters	= 1	dekaliter	10.0	grams	= 1	dekagram
100.0	liters	= 1	hectoliter	100.0	grams	= 1	hectogram
1000.0	liters	= 1	kiloliter	1000.0	grams	= 1	kilogram

Fig. 23-1 Metric units, divisions and multiples.

UNITS OF VOLUME					UNITS OF WEIGHT				
1	liter	=	1000	milliliters	1	gram	=	1000	milligrams
0.001	liter	=	1	milliliter	0.001	gram	=	1	milligram
				or					
	1			cubic centimeter	1	kilogram	=	1000	grams
					0.001	kilogram	=	1	gram

Fig. 23-2 Commonly used metric measurements.

used, physicians sometimes write the dose in words or Arabic numbers. CAUTION: The metric abbreviation for gram is gm; however, in the medical area, the abbreviation for gram (Gm) is usually capitalized to avoid confusion with grain (gr) which is not capitalized. The medical assistant must be aware of this fact and be very careful. *If the dose of any medication is not written clearly, she must not hesitate to ask the physician to verify it.*

Eventually, when the metric system is used predominantly, grains will be replaced by the gram or its equivalent fraction (15 grains equals 1 gram and 5 grains equals 0. 3 gram).

THE APOTHECARIES' SYSTEM

This system is still used extensively but is gradually being replaced by the metric system. The commonly used apothecary units must be memorized if the medical assistant is to administer medications and/or compute dosages, figure 23-3.

Abbreviations and Symbols

Frequently used symbols and abbreviations in the apothecaries' system are:

℥ or dr for dram   qt for quart

℥ or oz for ounce   O or pt for pint

♏ for minim   lb for pound

C or gal for gallon

In this system, Roman numerals are used when writing numbers of less than 100. Arabic numbers are used for numbers over 100, for fractions, and for mixed numbers. The abbreviation $\overline{ss}$ is used to indicate one-half. The following rules and examples will clarify the explanation:

- The symbol for the unit of measure is used; otherwise, the abbreviation may precede the number.

- The unit of measure is written *before* the number.

- The number is written in small Roman numerals.

- When using the Roman numeral one, a dot is placed over the number (i).

- A line is drawn over the numerals ($\overline{xv}$).

Example: The unit of measure is *dram.*

The abbreviation for dram is *dr*

The symbol for dram is ℥

Three drams may be written as ℥ⅲ

VOLUME					WEIGHT			
60	minims	= 1	(fluids)	dram	60	grains	= 1	dram
8	drams	= 1	(fluids)	ounce	8	drams	= 1	ounce
16	drams	= 1	pint		12	ounces	= 1	pound
2	pints	= 1	quart					

Fig. 23-3 Apothecary measurements.

VOLUME EQUIVALENTS		WEIGHT EQUIVALENTS	
METRIC	**APOTHECARIES'**	**METRIC**	**APOTHECARIES'**
1 milliliter	= 15 or 16 minims	0.06 gram or 60 milligrams	= 1 grain
4 milliliters	= 1 dram	1 gram or 1000 milligrams	= 15 grains
30 milliliters	= 1 ounce	500 milligrams	= 7½ grains
500 milliliters	= 1 pint	4 grams	= 1 dram
1000 milliliters	= 1 quart	30 grams	= 1 ounce

Fig. 23-4 Equivalency Chart for Volume and Weights.

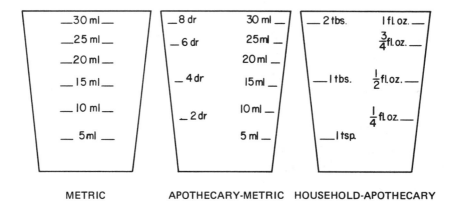

METRIC   APOTHECARY-METRIC   HOUSEHOLD-APOTHECARY

Fig. 23-5 Medicine cups.

Example: The unit of measure is *grain.*

The abbreviation for grain is *gr*

There is no symbol for *grain*

Ten grains may be written as gr x̄

APPROXIMATE EQUIVALENTS

To be able to work in both the metric and apothecaries' systems, the assistant must be able to convert from one system to the other. Conversion will result in an answer that is not an equal answer but an *equivalent answer;* this is an approximate answer, not an exact equal. The equivalents should be learned, figure 23-4.

NOTE: A milliliter and a cubic centimeter are accepted as equivalents. Medication cups are available in all of the systems but the medical assistant must concentrate on the metric and practice converting doses to metric, figure 23-5.

SUMMARY

There are two systems of measurement that are used in administering medications and computing their dosage. The metric system is the most accurate, flexible, and the easiest to use. This is the international system, and the United States is in the process of converting to it. However, the apothecaries' system is still in use at this time. The assistant must learn it and be able to convert from the metric to the apothecaries' system and vice versa. Conversion results in figures that are equivalent but not necessarily equal. The metric, apothecary, and approximate equivalent tables must be memorized.

SUGGESTED ACTIVITIES

- After memorizing the tables, have verbal quizzes (like a spelling bee) with the class divided equally and each student being eliminated for a wrong answer given.

- Visit a clinical laboratory and inspect some measurement devices, such as medicine glasses, graduated cylinders, gram scales, and rulers that are measured in both the metric and the apothecaries' system.

- Discuss the advantages of learning the metric system of weights and measures while in elementary school and using it in the mathematics departments of elementary schools.

REVIEW

1. Fill in the following blanks, using Arabic numbers and/or decimal fractions.

a. 1 mg	= _____ Gm		k.	oz. 2	= _____ ml
b. 2 ml	= _____ L		l.	gr. v	= _____ mg
c. 0.005 Gm	= _____ mg		m.	gr. s̄s̄	= _____ mg
d. 10 Gm	= _____ mg		n.	oz. 1 1/2	= _____ ml
e. 16 mg	= _____ Gm		o.	gr. 30	= _____ Gm
f. 500 mg	= _____ Gm		p.	dr. 2	= _____ ml
g. 2.25 Gm	= _____ mg		q.	gr. 7 1/2	= _____ mg
h. gr. 30	= _____ Gm		r.	oz. 1	= _____ drams
i. 0.1 Gm	= _____ gr		s.	dr. 1	= _____ minims
j. 1 1/2 ml	= _____ minims		t.	dr. 8	= _____ ml

Unit 24 Computation of Dosage

OBJECTIVES

After studying this unit, the student should be able to

- Differentiate between ratio and proportion.
- Compute dosage if the following cases are given:
  - a. If the dose ordered is the same as the dose on hand.
  - b. If the dose ordered is larger or smaller than the dose on hand.
  - c. If the dose ordered is in one system and the medicine on hand is in another system.
  - d. If the drug is in solution and the dose ordered is larger or smaller than the dose on hand.

In administering medications, the medical assistant will encounter situations where the drug ordered by the doctor is in one system of measurement and the drug on hand is labeled in another system. This creates a very real hazard. The assistant must be able to compute dosage in several different ways. This takes practice and absolute accuracy because a mistake could result in a loss of life.

RATIO AND PROPORTION

In addition to the terms and math related to the administration of medications, the medical assistant must thoroughly understand and be able to work with ratios and proportions. Ratios and proportions must be understood completely before continuing with computation of dosage.

A ratio indicates that there is a relationship between two numbers. Fractions are ratios, and ratios can be expressed as fractions. For example, 2/3 = 2:3 or 1:2 = 1/2.

A proportion is a statement indicating that two ratios are equivalent. For example, 1:25 = 2:50 (this is sometimes shown as 1:25 :: 2:50). The relationship between 1 and 25 is the same as that between 2 and 50.

All *true proportions* will have one thing in common: The product of the means will equal the product of the extremes. For example, in the proportion 1:25 = 2:50, the numbers 25 and 2 are the means and their product is 50. (25 x 2 = 50). The numbers, 1 and 50 are the extremes and their product is 50 (1 x 50 = 50) Therefore, 50 = 50. This is a true proportion. The following shows how to obtain a true proportion when one number is unknown (shown as X).

Example:

$$\overset{\text{means}}{X:4} = \overset{}{8:16} \qquad \text{Proof}$$
$$\underset{\text{extremes}}{} \qquad (X:4 \;=\; 8:16)$$

X16 = 4 x 8	2:4 = 8:16
16X = 32	2 x 16 = 4 x 8
X = 32 ÷ 16	32 = 32
X = 2	

By using the method of proof illustrated above, computations can be checked for accuracy.

COMPUTING DOSAGES

Situations which require knowledge about computing drugs usually fall in the following five categories (A-E).

A. If the doctor orders a dose of medicine and it is the same as the dosage on hand, there is no computation necessary.

Example: The doctor orders codeine phosphate gr s̄s̄ and the dose on hand is gr s̄s̄. One tablet would be given.

B. If the dose ordered by the doctor is in milligrams and the dose on hand is in grams, or vice versa, the dosage must be computed.

Example:

Ordered: 0.008 Gm
On hand: 16 mg tablets

The grams and milligrams must be converted to the same unit, then computed. Since 16 mg tablets are on hand and 0.008 *grams* have been ordered, it will be necessary to *convert the dosage from grams to milligrams and then determine how many or what part of the tablet must be given:*

- Convert to the same unit. (Refer to fig. 23-2, if necessary).
  Gm:mg = Gm:mg
  $0.001:1 = 0.008:X$

  $X = 8$ (means times extremes $= 8$)
  $X = 8$ mg (the dose ordered, converted to milligrams.)

  Remember, the proportion must be set up to see how much of the tablet (0.008 Gm) is to be given.

- Determine amount to be given.

mg:mg = tablet:tablet   Gm:Gm = tablet:tablet

$8:16 = X:1$	OR	$.008:.016 = X:1$
$16X = 8$		$8:16 = X:1$
$X = 1/2$ tablet		$16X = 8$
		$X = 8/16$
		$X = 1/2$ tablet

Practice Problems

1. How many tablets (or fractional parts) would be given in the following cases?

Enter final answer on line after *showing calculations.*

a. The doctor orders Diuril 0. 5 Gm. Only 250 mg tablets are on hand. Give ____ tablet(s).

b. Codeine sulfate 0.03 Gm tablets are on hand but the doctor orders 15 mg. Give _____ tablet(s).

c. The doctor orders Benadryl 50 mg. Capsules available are 0.025 Gm. Give _____ capsule(s).

C. If the doctor orders a dose of medicine that is larger or smaller than the dose that is on hand, the proportion would be as follows:

Example:

Ordered : gr 1/4
On hand : 1 tablet = gr 1/2

gr:gr = tablet:tablet   gr:tablets = gr:tablets

$1/4:1/2 = X:1$		$1/2:1 = 1/4:X$
$1/2X = 1/4$		$1/2X = 1/4$
$X = 1/4 \div 1/2$	OR	$X = 1/4 \div 1/2$
$X = 1/4 \times 2/1$		$X = 1/4 \times 2/1$
$X = 1/2$ tablet		$X = 1/2$ tablet

Practice Problems

2. How many tablets (or fractional parts) would be given in the following cases? Enter final answer on line after *showing calculations.*

a. The doctor orders Gantrisin 2 Gm. Tablets 0.5 Gm are on hand. Give _____ tablet(s).

b. Morphine 5 mg is ordered. Only 15 mg tablets are on hand. Give _____ tablet(s).

c. The doctor orders aspirin gr x̄. Only gr v̄ tablets are on hand. Give _____ tablet(s).

D. If the doctor orders a dose in one system but the medicine on hand is in another system, the correct dosage must be computed.

Example:

Ordered   : gr 1/150
On hand   : 1 tablet = Gm 0.0006

- Convert to the same unit. (.06 gram equals 1 grain). Refer to the preceding unit if necessary.

  Gm:gr = Gm:gr

  .06:1   = X:1/150
  X   = 1/150 x .06
  X   = .0004 Gm

- Now find how many tablets are to be given.

gr:tablet = gr:tablet   Gm:tablet = Gm:tablet

1/100:1 = 1/150:X   .0006:1 = .0004:X
1/100X = 1/150 OR .0006X = .0004
X = 1/150 ÷ 1/100   X = .0004 ÷ .0006
X = 1/150 x 100/1   X = 2/3 tablet
X = 2/3 tablet

Practice Problems

3. How many tablets or capsules would be given? Show calculations and indicate answer on the line.

   a. The doctor orders gr s̄s̄. Tablets 0.015 Gm are on hand. Give _____ tablet(s).

   b. The doctor orders 100 mg. Only capsules gr 5/6 are on hand. Give _____ capsule(s).

   c. The doctor orders gr ī. Only 30 mg tablets are on hand. Give _____ tablet(s).

E. If the doctor orders a drug that comes in solution form (diluted), it may be necessary to compute the dosage.

Example:

Ordered   : 25 mg
On hand : 5 mg per ml

- To determine how much is to be given, the proportion method may be used:

  mg:ml   =   mg:ml
  5:1   =   25:X
  5X   =   25
  X   =   5 ml to be given

If the dose is ordered in one system but what is on hand is in another system, the medical assistant must convert them both to the same unit or system.

Example:

Ordered : 0.5 Gm
On hand : 100 mg per ml

- Convert grams to milligrams (0. 5 Gm = 500 mg) or milligrams to grams (100 mg = 0.1 Gm). Then proceed as follows:

mg:ml	=	mg:ml		Gm:ml	=	Gm:ml
100:1	=	500:X		0.1:1	=	0.5:X
100X	=	500	OR	0.1X	=	0.5
X	=	5 ml		X	=	5 ml

Practice Problems

4. How much would be given in the following cases? Enter final answer on line after showing calculations.

    a. The doctor orders gr s̄s̄. The drug on hand is gr 1/4 in 4 ml. Give _____ ml.

b. The doctor orders gr x̄v̄. The drug on hand is gr v̄ in 1 dram. Give _____ drams.

c. The doctor orders 0.5 Gm. The drug on hand is gr x̄v̄ in 8 ml. Give _____ ml.

SUMMARY

The medical assistant must learn to do computation of dosage without error. True proportion is used to solve computation problems.

There are several different types of problems that must be solved and the assistant must learn to solve all of them.

SUGGESTED ACTIVITIES

- Review Units 22 and 23.
- Practice proportion problems, if difficulty is encountered in computation of dosage.
- Review the following figures which were found in the preceding unit.

UNITS OF VOLUME		UNITS OF WEIGHT	
1 liter	= 1000 milliliters	1 gram	= 1000 milligrams
0.001 liter	= 1 milliliter	0.001 gram	= 1 milligram
	or		
	1 cubic centimeter	1 kilogram	= 1000 grams
		0.001 kilogram	= 1 gram

VOLUME EQUIVALENTS			WEIGHT EQUIVALENTS		
METRIC		APOTHECARIES'	METRIC		APOTHECARIES'
1 milliliter	=	15 or 16 minims	0.06 gram or 60 milligrams	=	1 grain
4 milliliters	=	1 dram	1 gram or 1000 milligrams	=	15 grains
30 milliliters	=	1 ounce	500 milligrams	=	7½ grains
500 milliliters	=	1 pint	4 grams	=	1 dram
1000 milliliters	=	1 quart	30 grams	=	1 ounce

REVIEW

Solve the following problems.

1. Ordered: gr 1/2 On hand: 0.015 Gm tablets.   Give _____ .

2. Ordered: gr 1/32   On hand: 4 mg tablets.   Give _____ .

3. Ordered: 0.6 mg On hand: gr 1/100 tablets. Give _____ .

4. Ordered: 0.005 Gm   On hand: gr 1/4 tablets. Give _____ .

5. Ordered: gr 1 1/2 On hand: gr 1/2 tablets. Give _____ .

6. Ordered: 0.03 Gm On hand: gr 1/4 per dram. Give _____ .

7. Ordered: 0.4 mg On hand: gr 1/100 tablets. Give _____ .

8. Ordered: gr x̄x̄x̄ On hand: 1.0 Gm tablets.   Give _____ .

9. Ordered: 60 mg On hand: gr i tablets. Give _____ .

10. Ordered: 0.0010 Gm On hand: gr 1/120 tablets. Give _____ .

Unit 25 Classification of Drugs

OBJECTIVES

After studying this unit, the student should be able to

- Identify the action of each classification of drugs.
- Give an example of each drug classification.
- List the information that must be recorded on narcotic records.

The medical assistant must know how drugs are classified and how they act. This information includes individual drugs as well as general classifications. Drugs must not be given until this knowledge has been acquired.

STIMULANTS

A *stimulant* is a drug that increases the activities of the body or any of its individual organs. Stimulants increase the speed and strength of the heart action as well as the rate of respirations, digestive processes, and circulation.

There are many drugs that are classified as stimulants. **Caffeine** (caffeine sodium benzoate) is a commonly used stimulant. It raises blood pressure, increases circulation, increases respirations, strengthens the heartbeat, and increases the amount of urine produced (known as diuretic action). Each cup of coffee contains from 1 to 3 grains of caffeine, which is a central nervous system (CNS) stimulant, figure 25-1. **Epinephrine** (adrenalin) is a frequently used stimulant. *Amphetamines* are adrenergic drugs that affect the autonomic nervous system (ANS), figure 25-2, page 144. **Dexedrine** is an example of an amphetamine.

Some drugs primarily affect the mental state. These drugs are called antidepressants; they serve as mood elevators. They are most often used to relieve depression. **Elavil** is an example of an antidepressant drug.

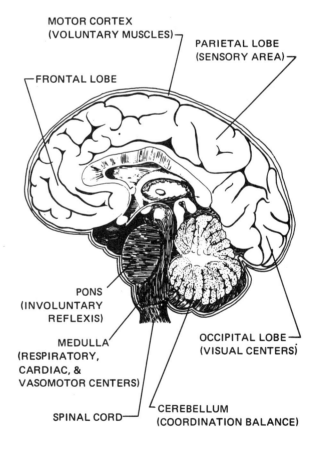

Fig. 25-1 The Central Nervous System.

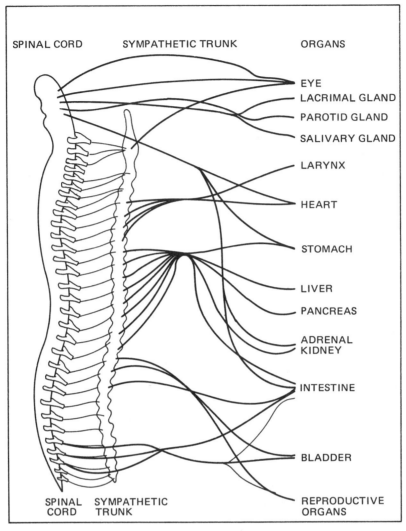

Fig. 25-2 The Autonomic Nervous System.

Stimulant drugs are not as numerous as the depressant drugs and, therefore, do not have as many different classifications.

DEPRESSANTS

There are many depressants on the market, many of which are *synthetically* produced; they are man made, produced artificially. *Depressants* decrease the body's activities. The heart function, respirations, digestive processes, and circulation are slowed by depressants. *Narcotics* or pain-killing medications are depressant in action. Drugs such as **opium** and some of its derivatives are narcotics that are obtained from a plant source. Narcotics relieve pain and cause the pupils of the eyes to contract. **Demerol** is a synthetic narcotic that is also a depressant.

Vasodilators such as **Nitroglycerin** dilate blood vessels and lower the blood pressure. Due to its action upon coronary blood vessels and the heart, it relieves the pain in a condition called angina pectoris. Nitroglycerin is administered sublingually.

Sedatives fall under the category of depressants. They are drugs that calm and quiet the patient so that he is more relaxed. Sedatives are not the same as tranquilizers although some of the actions produced are similar. Sedatives are used to produce a state of relaxation and sleep in the patient by slowing down the body functions. Most of the bromides fall into this category. **Glutethimide (Doriden)** is one of the orally effective sedatives.

Hypnotics are used to induce sleep. They do not relieve pain or serve as tranquilizers. They are prescribed solely to produce sleep in patients. Some sedatives and barbiturates are also hypnotics. *Barbiturates* depress the sleep centers of the brain and the motor areas. They also act on other parts of the central nervous system, and can cause death if taken in large doses. **Nembutal** and **seconal** are two examples of hypnotics that are classified as barbiturates. **Placidyl** is a nonbarbiturate hypnotic.

Some barbiturates are also used as *anticonvulsive* drugs. **Phenobarbital** is a barbiturate used as an anticonvulsive drug. (**Dilantin sodium** is an anticonvulsive drug which is *not* a barbiturate).

Tranquilizers reduce or lower the anxiety level of tense patients and allow agitated or disturbed people to relax and function in a calm, more normal manner. Tranquilizers are sometimes called *ataraxics*. They are frequently used in the treatment of mentally disturbed patients and in conjunction with psychotherapy. Even though they do not produce drowsiness or sleep, many tranquilizers are habit-forming and dangerous. They must be used with great care to avoid addiction in dependent patients. **Meprobamate, Promazine,** and **Chlorpromazine** are some commonly used tranquilizers.

Anticholinergic drugs are also depressants. They depress the response of the autonomic nervous system. They are also responsible for decreasing peristalsis (intestinal movements), bladder contractions, and secretions such as saliva, bronchial and intestinal secretions. **Atropine sulfate** is a frequently used anticholinergic. It is often given before surgery.

to dry up secretions which the patient might otherwise aspirate while under anesthesia.

Analgesics relieve pain. They range from a mild to a very strong effect. Aspirin is a mild analgesic. It is also used as an *antipyretic* (fever reducing drug). Many drugs are available to the public without a prescription. These drugs are the milder analgesics. Many of them are *patent medicines* which means they are sold without prescription. The pain-killing narcotics discussed earlier are considered very strong analgesics; **Morphine** is an example.

OTHER CLASSIFICATIONS OF DRUGS

Some categories of drugs are better classified in groups other than stimulants or depressants.

Antihistamines are drugs that cut down on the production of secretions and relieve allergic conditions. They are effective in relieving the discomforts caused by allergies, nasal congestion due to colds, hayfever, and sinusitis. **Chlorpheniramine maleate (Teldron)** is a commonly used antihistamine.

Antibiotics are drugs that are given to destroy pathogenic organisms in the body. **Penicillin** is probably the best known of the antibiotics. Originally the antibiotics were produced by molds but are now made synthetically. There are many antibiotics available today for various types of pathogens (disease-causing organisms). However, some people are allergic to antibiotics. Always ask if the patient is allergic to antibiotics, if a skin test has not been done, before administering any antibiotics.

Anticoagulants are another group of drugs that are potentially dangerous for the patient. Anticoagulants slow the blood-clotting process. They may be prescribed when patients form blood clots that obstruct blood vessels. Whenever anticoagulants are given, there is a distinct danger that the patient's blood may lose the ability to clot at all. This could result in a great loss of blood from internal or external hemorrhage. Blood tests are done routinely when anticoagulants are given. **Coumadin sodium** is an anticoagulant.

Antidiarrheals are drugs given to stop diarrhea. **Kaolin** and **kaopectate** are antidiarrheals.

Cathartics are drugs that have a laxative action. They cause the intestines to evacuate. **Milk of magnesia** and **mineral oil** are used to cause or facilitate bowel movements.

Emetics are drugs that induce vomiting. They are used in cases where vomiting is necessary to empty the stomach contents. Ingestion of large amounts of alcohol will sometimes cause acute alcohol poisoning. **Syrup of Ipecac** is occasionally used to induce vomiting and is a powerful emetic.

Expectorants either increase or decrease the secretions of mucous membranes that line the respiratory tract. They are given to reduce coughing. **Sodium iodide** and **potassium iodide** increase bronchial secretions which dilutes the thick sputum and enables the patient to cough it up. **Terpin hydrate** decreases secretions and affects the cough center of the brain, thereby, suppressing the cough.

Hormones influence the balance of the glandular secretions in the body. There are many types of hormonal drugs and they are given for a multitude of reasons. An example is **Premarin** which is given to lessen the discomforts of menopause. Some hormones are also used in the treatment of various kinds of cancer.

Vitamins are preparations that are used to supplement deficient diets but can also be used to treat disease conditions. Vitamin K is used to treat conditions that cause excessive bleeding and poor blood clotting. Ulcerative colitis is sometimes treated with Vitamin K.

DRUG LEGISLATION

The United States has had laws designed to protect the consumers since 1906;

at that time the Pure Food Act was passed. In 1937, over a hundred people died as a result of ingestion of a drug. As a result, the law was amended and in 1938 it became the Federal Food, Drug, and Cosmetic Act.

Since 1938, there have been several amendments designed to better protect the consumer. In 1952, the Durham-Humphrey Law tightened the controls on barbiturates and set regulations for refills of barbiturate drugs.

The Harrison Narcotic Act, originally passed in 1914 but amended several times, has regulated the control of narcotics for many years. All people handling or dealing with narcotics must be registered with the Depart- of Internal Revenue. Detailed records are kept of all narcotics. The registered physician prescribes narcotics and a registered pharmacist fills the prescription. If a nurse or assistant administers a narcotic, a detailed record must be kept. These records are inspected at intervals by the Department of Internal Revenue. The following information is recorded:

- Patient's name.
- Name of the drug.
- Dosage given.
- Route of administration.
- Date drug is given.
- Name of the person administering the drug.

In 1970, the Harrison Narcotic Law was replaced by the Controlled Substance Act which contains substantially the same regulations and covers some non-narcotic drugs. The assistant must know what drugs are controlled by federal legislation. The local library will be able to supply the name of the department to contact for copies of the law.

All drugs are dangerous when handled carelessly or when taken or administered without full knowledge of the action of the drug and its consequences. Death can result from drug abuse.

SUMMARY

Drugs are classified as depressants (which include several subclassifications), stimulants, and other miscellaneous categories. The medical assistant must know the classification and action of the drugs she administers. Drugs are dangerous and must be handled with knowledge and respect.

There are several laws that control and regulate drugs. All records maintained for the Department of Internal Revenue must be accurate, up-to-date, and contain all information required. The assistant will be responsible for these records.

SUGGESTED ACTIVITIES

- Review current pharmacology texts for information about drug legislation.

- Make arrangements to invite a physician to give a lecture on drug abuse. Request time for a question-and-answer session.

- Begin a drug card library for your personal use. Keep a 5 x 7 index card on each drug. Write the generic name, trade name, usual dosage given, usual method of administration, indications, and contraindications of the drug. Write a brief description of the action of the drug at the bottom of the card. Store all cards in an index box for quick and easy access.

REVIEW

A. Match the following drugs with the proper classification.

1. _____ hormone	a. adrenalin
2. _____ emetic	b. terpin hydrate
3. _____ anticoagulant	c. kaolin
4. _____ barbiturate	d. caffeine
5. _____ sedative	e. chlorpheniramine maleate
6. _____ antidiarrheal	
7. _____ antidepressant	f. Syrup of Ipecac
8. _____ expectorant	g. premarin
9. _____ antihistamine	h. penicillin
10. _____ antibiotic	i. aspirin
11. _____ CNS stimulant	j. atropine sulfate
12. _____ anticonvulsive barbiturate	k. milk of magnesia
13. _____ tranquilizer	l. morphine
14. _____ anticholinergic	m. coumadin sodium
15. _____ cathartic	n. chlorpromazine
16. _____ narcotic	o. placidyl
17. _____ antipyretic	p. dilantin sodium
18. _____ nonbarbiturate hypnotic	q. doriden
19. _____ nonbarbiturate anticonvulsive	r. nembutal
	s. elavil
20. _____ ANS stimulant	t. phenobarbital

B.   Match the classification of drug with the action.

1. _____ reduces the anxiety level.
2. _____ depresses the sleep centers and motor areas of the brain.
3. _____ relieves pain.
4. _____ decreases peristalsis, bladder contractions, and secretions.
5. _____ reduces or suppresses coughing.
6. _____ increases production of urine.
7. _____ used to produce a state of relaxation.
8. _____ produces sleep.
9. _____ produces laxative effect.
10. _____ destroys pathogenic organisms.
11. _____ supplements a deficient diet.
12. _____ relieves allergic conditions such as nasal congestion.
13. _____ mood elevators.
14. _____ induces vomiting.
15. _____ reduces clotting time.
16. _____ influences the hormonal chemical balance of the body.
17. _____ reduces fever.
18. _____ stops diarrhea.
19. _____ increases body activities.
20. _____ decreases body activities.

a. analgesic
b. hypnotic
c. tranquilizer
d. expectorant
e. diuretic
f. depressant
g. sedative
h. hormone
i. cathartic
j. vitamin
k. antihistamine
l. anticholinergic
m. barbiturates
n. emetic
o. anticoagulant
p. antidepressant
q. stimulant
r. antibiotic
s. antipyretic
t. antidiarrheal

C.   List the information that must be recorded on narcotic records.

Unit 26 Principles of Drug Administration

OBJECTIVES

After studying this unit, the student will be able to

- State the rules and precautions for administering medications.
- List the methods of administrations and give the reasons.
- Cite the state law governing drug administration by medical assistants.

The medical assistant may be required at times to administer medications to patients. She must learn and abide by the principles or rules for administration of medication.

GENERAL PRINCIPLES

All drugs are potentially dangerous; the assistant is responsible for all medications that she gives to patients. There are rules for administering any medications:

- **Full attention must be given to preparation and administration of all medications at all times.**
- **All orders for medications are noted on the patient's record.**
- **Administration of medication must be recorded: the time the drug was given, the method of administration, the dosage, and patient reaction, if any.**

- **All medication notations on patient records must be dated and initialed.**
- **All drug labels are checked and compared with the order three times before giving any drug. Labels are checked:**
  a. upon removal from the cabinet
  b. before pouring the medication
  c. before replacing container in the cabinet
- **No drug is ever returned to its container after it has been removed. It must be discarded if not used.**
- *Always ask the patient if he is allergic to any drugs before giving any medications.* Patients have died from drug reactions.
- **Always keep drug cabinets and storage areas for drugs locked.**
- **Always give the patient sufficient amounts of water to take with oral med-**

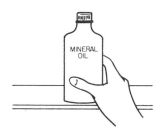 1. Removing from cabinet.

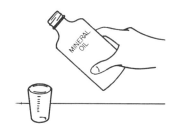 2. Before pouring.

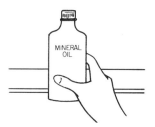 3. Before replacing in cabinet.

Fig. 26-1 Read the label 3 times.

ications. A paper cup is used for this purpose. It is poor practice to expect a patient to take oral medications at a water fountain. It is also dangerous since choking and aspiration can occur if the medication blocks the air passages.

- All narcotics must be recorded on a special narcotic sheet that will be checked by federal narcotics agents at unannounced intervals.

- Liquids are always poured at eye level. Pour from the side of the bottle *away* from the label. The outside of the bottle must be kept clean; any excess liquid that might run down the side of the bottle is wiped off.

- Place thumbnail against the measurement line on the medication glass to assure accuracy of exact dose.

- If the doctor orders a drug to be given in the office, stay with the patient until the medicine has been swallowed. Always offer the medication in a medicine cup.

- The medical assistant must be familiar with all drugs that she administers. She must know what the usual dosage is and what the contraindications (situations where it would not be given) are. If unfamiliar with the drug being given, it should be looked up in the drug reference books in the office.

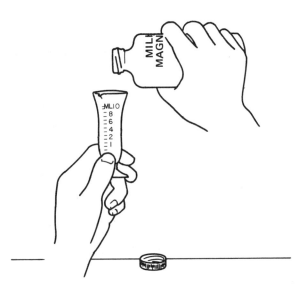

Fig. 26-2 Pouring a liquid at eye level with label up and thumbnail held at point on amount needed.

Handling drugs requires a great amount of responsibility. No drug is harmless. Children and adults have died from taking plain aspirin. Drugs are never given or recommended by the assistant *except by express order from the physician.*

RESPONSIBILITIES

The medical assistant should contact the State Education Department or the local library to learn about state laws governing drug administration by medical assistants. She is also responsible for ordering, storing, and record keeping of the medications. She must be very diligent in all these responsibilities if she is to be trusted with drugs.

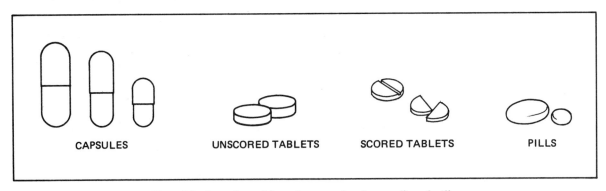

Fig. 26-3 Capsules, tablets (unscored and scored) and pills.

Too many unnecessary tragedies have happened in the past due to carelessness of the people administering medications. There is never any excuse for medication errors or accidents. The medical assistant assumes responsibility for the patient's health when administering medications. Absolute accuracy and concentration is necessary for anyone handling medications.

Poisons are always kept separately from other medications. Labels must always be legible. Unlabeled bottles are thrown away. Drugs that require refrigeration should be kept refrigerated at all times to preserve the effectiveness of the drug.

Do not overstock medications; the chemical elements in drugs may break down and change if kept too long. Expiration dates should be noted and drugs should never be used beyond that date. Always store drugs in a cabinet that is not accessible to the patients. Keep all drug areas spotlessly clean. Cabinets must be wiped down with a cleaning solution at weekly intervals.

The doctor writes the medication order and the medical assistant refers to it when medicine is to be given to a patient.

NOTE: If for any reason, the doctor gives a verbal order, the medical assistant must immediately write down the order and the doctor's instructions before she gives the medication. This serves several purposes:

- The right patient receives the right medication.

- The name of the drug, the dosage and the route of administration are verified.

- It serves as a reliable check to ensure correct notations on the patient's record.

- If the medicine cannot be given promptly or if the physician is to give the drug, the written instructions can serve as a label until the drug is administered.

Remember to look up new medications before administering them to the patient.

METHODS OF ADMINISTRATION

In addition to oral administration, there are other methods of giving medications:

- parenterally (injection)

- inunction (topically)

- sublingually (under the tongue)

- internal insertion (suppositories)

- inhalation

Medication may be given *parenterally* (by injection) rather than orally for several reasons. Frequently medications are given by injection because a faster response is desired. Of course, the absorption rate of the drug will affect how quickly a response is achieved. At times, it is advisable to give drugs parenterally because the patient may be having nausea and vomiting which would make it impossible for him to retain the drug if taken orally. Also, some drugs are adversely affected by the gastric juices in the stomach and will be altered or destroyed if taken into the digestive tract. Other medications may cause nausea and vomiting if taken orally; gastric upset can be avoided by parenteral administration of these drugs.

When a drug is given by injection, the exact dosage is controlled. Also, it is certain that the patient has received the drug. This is not always true if the patient must take the drug orally. The effects of drugs are more reliable and results are often more prompt and complete when they are received by injection.

Drugs may also be administered by *inunction* or *topically*. This means that drugs may be applied to the skin in the form of an ointment or a liquid, as in the case of topical anesthesia.

Occasionally, tablets are ordered to be given *sublingually*. When this happens, the medication is placed under the tongue for dissolving and absorption. Nitroglycerin, a com-

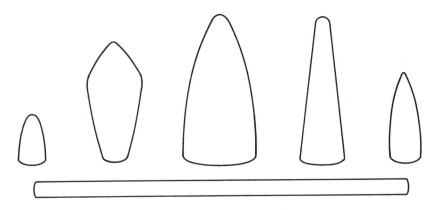

Fig. 26-4 Suppositories: urethral, vaginal and rectal.

mon medication for high blood pressure, is administered sublingually.

Medications may be inserted *internally* into a body cavity as in the case of suppositories. Suppositories are small amounts of medication contained in a substance that melts at body temperature; the drug is released and is absorbed into the mucous membranes of the rectum, vagina, or urethra.

Inhalation is another method of administration of medications but one that is not used often in the doctor's office. However, the doctor may request that the patient use the inhalation method at home; this is usually done by adding an inhalant medication to a vaporizer or steam kettle. *The medication is not to be taken internally!* It is greatly diluted by the water vapor and steam and is taken in through the respiratory system.

Regardless of the method of administration, all medications must be treated with great care and respect. The rules for administration of medications must be followed carefully and at all times. There is no room for mistakes where a patient's life is concerned. When in doubt ask the physician. *The medical assistant must always be sure she is giving the ordered medication to the correct patient and that the dose is accurately administered.*

SUMMARY

There are certain rules for preparation and administration of medications which must be followed at all times. Full, undivided attention must be given to the preparation and administration of all drugs.

There are several methods of administration: oral, parenteral, inunction or topical, sublingual, internal insertion, and inhalation. The assistant must be familiar with all drugs that she gives. A clear, complete, and concise report of the medication, its dosage, its route or administration, the date, time, and the medical assistant's initials are charted immediately after the medication is given. Any reaction the patient has is also recorded.

SUGGESTED ACTIVITIES

- Look up the following drugs in one of the drug manuals. List the action of the drug, its usual dosage, routes of administration, contraindications, and effectiveness.

<table>
<tr><td>Digitalis</td><td>Morphine</td></tr>
<tr><td>Compazine</td><td>Adrenalin</td></tr>
<tr><td>Ampicillin</td><td>Demerol</td></tr>
</table>

- Using outside resources, define *trade name* and *generic name.*
- Practice following a doctor's order for administration of an oral medication. Use medicine cups, pour out the "medications" and follow the steps given in this unit. Role play these techniques with fellow students; with the instructor's guidance, check and evaluate them.

REVIEW

1. After administering medications, what information is recorded on the patient record?

2. List the three times a label is read.

3. How are liquids poured from a bottle? Why?

4. In addition to administering medications, name three other responsibilities the medical assistant has regarding medications.

5. Give four reasons for writing down the doctor's instructions about medications to be given.

6. List five methods of administration other than orally.

7. Why are labels read three times before giving a medication?

8. If a drug has been prepared for use but not given, what should be done with it?

9. Why must the medical assistant stay with the patient when giving medications?

10. Why should the medical assistant take the time to look up a drug in the drug book before giving it?

11. What should be remembered about storing poisons?

12. What does your state law say about drug administration by medical assistants?

Unit 27 Injections

OBJECTIVES

After studying this unit, the student should be able to

- List the types of injections and the most commonly used injection sites for each.
- Relate the reasons for giving medication by injection.
- State the dangers of injections.

Injections are given subcutaneously, intramuscularly, intravenously, or intradermally.

CAUTION: These injections are given only if the medical assistant has had instruction and practice. Also, the medical assistant never gives any medication without permission to administer the medication.

The medical assistant may have to learn how to administer injections except by the intravenous method.

Anytime an injection is given, two foreign objects are introduced into the patient's tissues: the needle and the drug. Great care must be taken to see that this procedure is carried out under aseptic technique. Knowing the proper site for the injection is also very important.

REASONS FOR INJECTIONS

There are several reasons for giving medication by the injection method rather than one of the other routes of administration.

It is sometimes necessary to obtain an immediate effect, so a drug is given by injection instead of by the oral method. The injection method results in immediate action as the drug reaches the bloodstream more quickly.

In some instances, a patient may not be able to take the medication orally, or it may not be safe to use this route. The mental or physical state of the patient could prohibit oral medications. Also, some drugs cannot be given orally because of their chemical composition and the action of the drug on mucous membranes. Digestive juices may also alter the action of the drug.

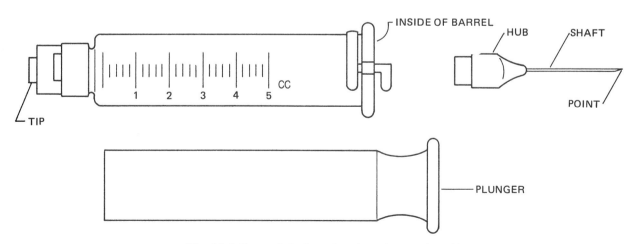

Fig. 27-1 Parts of the hypodermic syringe and needle.

If the drug is given *parenterally,* or by injection, the exact amount of drug that is acting is controlled. A local reaction may be obtained with hypodermic injections of a drug that would not be possible with other methods of administration. For example, local anesthesia may be given by a hypodermic to carry out a procedure on a small area. A general anesthesia would not be necessary.

DANGERS OF INJECTIONS

Unfortunately, there are some serious dangers involved in the administration of injections. Perhaps the greatest danger is that this is a routine, common procedure; people often tend to become careless when carrying out a routine procedure.

The assistant must recognize these dangers and recognize that even though the procedure is routine, it must be carried out carefully and with complete concentration and knowledge.

There is also the danger of causing injury or damage to the patient when drugs are given by injection. An injection can result in injury to blood vessels, superficial nerves, or even other anatomical structures if the assistant does

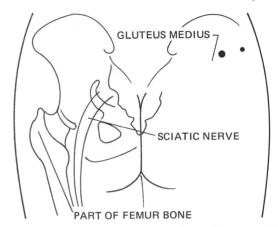

Fig. 27-2 **Select the proper site for an intramuscular injection to avoid injury to blood vessels, nerves and other structures.**

not thoroughly understand anatomy as well as proper site location technique, figure 27-2.

Needles may break off in the patient's tissues if the assistant is not very careful. This is an acute danger with children who are frightened and are difficult to give injections.

Development of an abcess is possible any time a foreign object is introduced into tissues; this is also true of injections. Abcesses may be the results of:

- Improper sterilization or disinfection of the injection site.

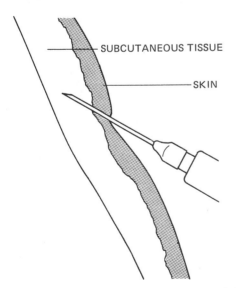
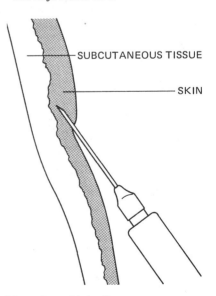

Fig. 27-3 **Subcutaneous injection and Intradermal injection.**

- Use of needle or syringe that was not properly cleaned and sterilized.

- Unclean hands giving the injection.

- Injecting a drug where it cannot be absorbed by the tissue.

NOTE: Injection of a drug into a vein rather than into the body tissues can result in very great danger to the patient. Drugs that are beneficial when absorbed by the tissue can be hazardous and even fatal if given in a vessel. This is the reason for *aspiration,* or checking to see that the needle is not in a vein. This is done by withdrawing the plunger (inner portion of the syringe) after piercing the skin and before discharging the contents of the syringe into the tissues.

TYPES OF INJECTIONS

The subcutaneous injection is the method used most frequently. The drug is "placed" in the subcutaneous tissue between the skin and the underlying muscles. The injection site chosen may be the upper, outer arm (deltoid area), the outer thigh (vastus lateralis area), or — in special instances — other specific areas of the body. The deltoid site is most often used. *Aqueous* solutions are given subcutaneously; this means the drug is dissolved in a water base solution. A 25-gauge needle is usually used and no more than 2 milliliters (2 cc) of solution is given subcutaneously.

Insulin syringes have scale markings according to standard unit strengths, usually U 40 or U 80. The needle used may be a 25-gauge, 5/8 inch length or a 26-gauge, 1/2 inch length.

The vial which contains the insulin shows how many units are contained in one cubic centimeter, that is, units 40 or units 80 in 1 cc. The strength determines what scale on the syringe will be used. For example, if the insulin on hand is U 40 and the doctor orders U 30, the U 40 syringe is used. *Never use a U 40*

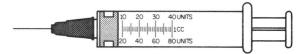

syringe to administer U 80 insulin and vice versa. Study the illustration of an insulin syringe.

The intradermal injection is used when the skin reaction to a given substance is being tested. Allergy tests and some other reaction determinations, such as the tuberculin skin test, are examples of the intradermal injection. Very short, small needles (26-gauge) are used for this method and only a tiny amount of medication is placed immediately under the surface of the skin. Allergy tests are usually administered by the doctor and readings made by him.

When medications are given intramuscularly, they are placed into the deep muscles such as the gluteus *medius.* This technique requires a greater knowledge and understanding of anatomy and physiology than does the subcutaneous injection as deeper tissue is invaded. Refer again to figure 27-2.

CAUTION: Never inject medication into the buttock (gluteus maximus).

A 20-gauge needle is used for thick, viscous solutions and a 21- or 22-gauge needle may be used for thinner substances. The needle must be at least one-inch long. Intramuscular injections are given for the following reasons:

- When large amounts of medication must be administered.

- When the substance given is an oil based solution or other substance which will cause tissue irritation.

- Some drugs cause strong reactions that are more easily tolerated in muscle tissue than subcutaneous tissue.

Intravenous injections are a method of placing a drug directly into the bloodstream (20-gauge needles are usually used.) *The doc-*

tor administers medication intravenously because of its great danger. However, the assistant may prepare the drug. This is a procedure that requires the greatest care in performing. The assistant must be certain of the action of the drugs she handles and must also be aware of the dangers involved in giving any drugs. Mistakes are fatal.

LOCAL ANESTHETICS

Local anesthetics are administered by injections in three ways. First is the subcutaneous method discussed earlier. The medication is injected directly into the tissues that are to be anesthetized. The second method is *intra-articular injection.* This means injecting the drug directly into a joint. The physician will carry out this procedure, but the assistant will prepare the setup. The third method is injection into the areas surrounding bony tissue, as in the case of fractures. The doctor may use this method to anesthetize a fracture enabling him to reduce the fracture without the use of a general anesthetic. It is often used in minor surgery.

The same procedure may be followed to remove a substance from the body as well as to inject a drug. For example, preparation for a lumbar puncture is based on the same principles as for injection administration; however, spinal fluid is removed instead of the injection of a drug. This procedure is performed by the doctor but preparation of the setup, supporting the patient emotionally and physically, and sending the *uncontaminated* fluid to the laboratory for studies may be part of the medical assistant's duties.

INJECTION PREPARATION

Due to the widespread usage of disposable hypodermic supplies, the danger of cross contamination between patients has been decreased. Sterile technique must still be followed but sterile disposable needles and syringes are much safer than the reusable ones. All disposable equipment is used ONCE then disposed of properly.

To set up or prepare for the administration of injections, the following equipment is needed:

- A small tray to hold the equipment.
- Sterile prepackaged hypodermic sets (syringe and needle).
- Sterile syringe of correct size (2 cc, 3 cc, 6 cc, etc.)

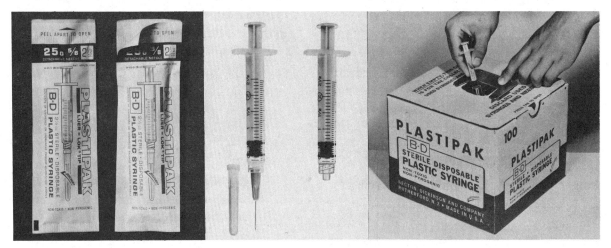

Fig. 27-4 Disposable sterile hypodermic set. The empty carton in which the hypodermic sets were packed, may be used to discard used sets.

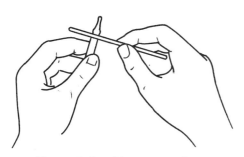

Fig. 27-5 Breaking an ampule.

- Sterile needle of correct size (25-gauge, 21-gauge, 20-gauge, etc.)

- Sterile sponges of prepackaged preparations to cleanse the skin (usually alcohol 70% prepackaged gauze sponges).

- Solution to be used for skin preparation if prepackaged skin preps are not used. (Alcohol 70%)

- The drug to be injected. (ABSOLUTELY STERILE!)

PROCEDURE

Contact with any unsterile object will contaminate a sterile object.

Preparing the Injection

The sterile disposable hypodermic set is removed from the paper wrapping. The needle is usually encased in a sterile, disposable, plastic sheath. Although the outside of the syringe and sheath become contaminated by handling, *care is taken not to contaminate the tip of the syringe,* review figure 27-1. (Sometimes, the sheath and needle may accidentally be pulled away from the tip of the syringe.)

If the separately packaged sterile syringes and sterile needles are used, the same principles regarding sterility apply. The desired needle (correct gauge size) is selected; it is in a plastic container with a plastic cap.

The needle is removed from its container by first removing the little cap; this cap covers the hub which will fit onto the separate sterile

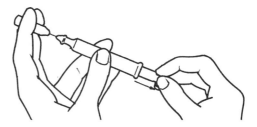

Fig. 27-6 Withdrawing solution from an ampule.

syringe. The protective covering for the shaft and point of the needle (the plastic sheath) remains in place until the drug has been drawn up into the syringe.

The drug may be contained in an ampule or a vial. If the medication is in an ampule, the medical assistant must be careful when inserting the needle in the ampule; the rim must not be touched with the needle or the needle will be contaminated.

A vial must be cleaned thoroughly by rubbing the rubber cap (that the needle passes through) with an alcohol sponge or cotton ball soaked in 70% alcohol. It is not touched with the fingers, only the sponge. The cap is removed from the needle and the syringe barrel is drawn back to the desired number of cubic centimeters. (This is not necessary with an open ampule). This action prevents a vacuum from forming and making it difficult to withdraw the solution from the vial. The drug is drawn into the syringe without air bubbles after carefully inserting the needle through the rubber cap. The needle and syringe are gently removed. The needle used to withdraw

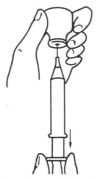

Fig. 27-7 Withdrawing solution from a vial (after air has been injected into vial).

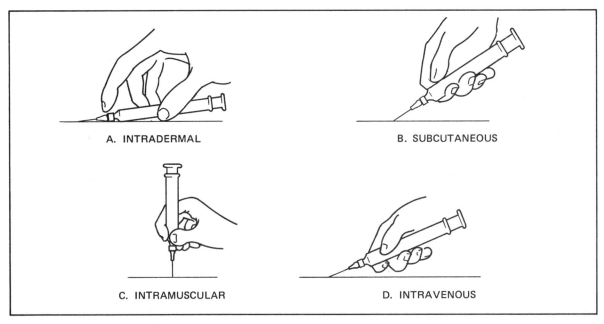

A. INTRADERMAL

B. SUBCUTANEOUS

C. INTRAMUSCULAR

D. INTRAVENOUS

Fig. 27-8 Angle of injections.

the medication is replaced by another sterile needle. The amount of medication and the label are checked again carefully.

Giving the Injection

Be sure to tell the patient that the medication ordered is to be given by injection. A sterile sponge with antiseptic is used to prepare the skin for injection. Again, 70% alcohol is commonly used for this purpose. The injection site is wiped in a circular motion from the center outward to remove dirt and germs from the area. If the medical assistant is right-handed, the muscle at the injection site is grasped with the left hand. Place the needle at the correct angle for entering the site (60° for subcutaneous, 90° for intramuscular) then quickly insert the needle into the tissue. Withdraw the plunger slightly to be sure the needle is not into a blood vessel.

CAUTION: No blood should enter the barrel of the syringe. If it does, the needle is in a vessel and should be removed immediately. After checking by this method (aspiration), the solution is slowly injected into the tissues. With the alcohol sponge held in the left hand

and held close to the arm, the needle is removed quickly. The injection site is massaged *gently* with the alcohol sponge. This helps to disperse the drug and relieve local discomfort.

Injection techniques must be practiced until the assistant can administer a quick, sure, accurate injection. A steady hand and confidence that comes through practice are necessary to give injections that cause the patient little or no discomfort.

SUMMARY

There are several methods of giving injections; sterile technique must be practiced with all methods. The subcutaneous and intramuscular methods will be used most often by the assistant. Only the doctor gives intravenous medications.

The assistant must be knowledgeable about the drugs she prepares and gives. The dangers involved in giving an injection must always be kept in mind even though it is a routine procedure. An understanding of human anatomy and physiology is necessary to give injections safely.

SUGGESTED ACTIVITIES

- Review the parts of the anatomy that are used as injection sites. Take careful note of the blood vessels and nerves that are located near the sites most frequently used.

- Under supervision, practice preparing injections in a sterile procedure, using water for injection. An orange may be used for the actual injection of the water to provide practice in inserting the needle and discharging the medication.

- Prepare a setup for a subcutaneous injection; intramuscular injection; intradermal injection; and intravenous injection. Have the instructor evaluate the activity.

REVIEW

A. Fill in the blanks with the correct type of injection.

1. _____ is given in the gluteus medius, vastus lateralis, or other deep muscles.

2. _____ usually given in the deltoid area, and it the most frequently given type of injection.

3. _____ is given between the surfaces of the skin and the underlying subcutaneous tissue. Used for skin testing.

4. _____ given directly into the bloodstream. Administered by the physician but often prepared by the assistant.

5. _____ injecting a drug directly into a joint. Done only by a physician.

6. _____ eliminates the need for a general anesthesia, used in minor surgery.

B. List four reasons why drugs may be given by a method other than oral administration.

1.
2.
3.
4.

C. Complete the following statements.

1. A specific procedure that is similar to the injection technique except that a fluid is removed rather than injected is the _____ .

2. Fill in the blank with the size of gauge needle that would be used in each situation.

    a. _____ A subcutaneous injection of less than 2 cc.

    b. _____ An intradermal injection for allergy testing.

    c. _____ An intravenous injection of a thick, viscous substance.

    d. _____ An intramuscular injection of an aqueous solution.

    e. _____ An intravenous injection of an aqueous solution.

    f. _____ An intramuscular injection of a thick, viscous substance.

3. Fill in the blanks with the correct word.

    a. _____ is the practice of withdrawing the plunger of the syringe a little bit after the needle is placed in the tissue. It is a check to be sure the needle is not in a blood vessel.

    b. _____ is most commonly used as a skin prep for the injection site. It may be prepackaged or used to soak sterile cotton balls.

    c. _____ needles and syringes are much safer than reusable ones because it eliminates cross contamination.

D. Circle the correct answer.

    1. If an intravenous injection is to be given

        a. the assistant will prepare and give it at the doctor's instruction.
        b. the physician will always prepare and administer the injection.
        c. the assistant may be asked to prepare the medication and the physician will give it.
        d. none of the above.

    2. Air is injected into a vial before withdrawing solution to

        a. be sure that it is sterile.
        b. prevent a vacuum from forming.
        c. act as a safety device.
        d. be sure the needle is open.

3. The injection site is cleaned with 70% alcohol by wiping the site in a

   a. up and down scrubbing motion.
   b. circular motion, covering the area at least twice.
   c. circular motion, using sterile forceps to hold the sponge securely.
   d. circular motion from the inside of the area to the outside.

4. The correct angle for entering the skin for an intramuscular injection is

   a. 75°
   b. 50°
   c. 90°
   d. 60°

5. Injection techniques must be practiced by the assistant until she can

   a. give an injection without any pain.
   b. give quick, sure, accurate injections.
   c. give all kinds of injections.
   d. do a, b, and c.

Self-Evaluation Test 4

Choose the answers that best complete the following statements.

1. Chemotherapy is the treatment of illness and injury using

   a. drugs.
   b. X rays.
   c. physical therapy.
   d. methods of heat.

2. Pharmacology is defined as

   a. the administration of drugs by anyone trained to give them.
   b. the treatment of disease using drugs.
   c. the science of drugs and their actions on the human body.
   d. substances that are used as medicines.

3. The correct abbreviation for the term which means immediately is

   a. subq.
   b. stat.
   c. NPO.
   d. ung.

4. The correct Roman numeral for number 50 is

   a. V.
   b. XXXXX.
   c. L.
   d. LC.

5. PRN is the abbreviation for the term

   a. three times a day.
   b. whenever necessary.
   c. hour of sleep.
   d. nothing by mouth.

6. A liter is a unit of measurement used in

   a. the apothecaries' system to measure fluid.
   b. the metric system to measure solid weight.
   c. the metric system to measure fluid volume.
   d. the apothecaries' system to measure length.

7. The approximate weight equivalent of one grain in the apothecaries' system is

   a. 15 minims in the apothecaries' system.
   b. 0.06 gram in the metric system.
   c. one dram in the apothecaries' system.
   d. 4 milliliters in the metric system.

8. If the doctor orders Atropine gr 1/150 to be given and 0.0002 gram tablets are on hand, how many tablet(s) would be given to administer gr 1/150?

   a. one tablet.
   b. one-half tablet.
   c. two tablets.
   d. 2/3 tablet.

9. The medical assistant may be responsible for

    a. administering medications. c. restocking the drug supply.
    b. storing drugs.   d. all of these.

10. If a drug has been prepared for administration but is not given, it is

    a. immediately discarded.
    b. put back into the container.
    c. set aside for possible use later.
    d. any of the three above, depending upon the circumstances.

11. Two of the following books are legal standard books for drugs in the United States. They are the

    a. Physician's Desk Reference.
    b. National Formulary.
    c. Pharmacopoeia of the United States of America.
    d. Pharmacopoeia Internationalis.

12. Medications are administered by injection because

    a. the composition of the drug makes it necessary.
    b. administration by injection is quicker.
    c. the exact amount administered is under control.
    d. all of the above.

13. Whenever a foreign substance or object is introduced into body tissue, there is a possibility of

    a. abcess formation.   c. bruising of the bone.
    b. profuse bleeding.   d. none of these.

14. The most frequently used method of injecting medication into the body is

    a. intramuscularly.   c. subcutaneously.
    b. intravenously.   d. intradermally.

15. The reason why the plunger of the syringe is withdrawn after an injection (aspiration) is to

    a. avoid injecting air into a vein.
    b. avoid injecting medication into a blood vessel.
    c. ensure that the needle is far enough into the tissues.
    d. ensure that the needle is not resting on a bone.

16. The gluteus medius muscle would most likely be used for administering an

    a. intramuscular injection.   c. intravenous injection.
    b. intradermal injection.   d. subcutaneous injection.

17. Air is injected into a vial before withdrawing the solution for injection to

    a. be sure that the lumen of the needle is open.
    b. avoid creating a vacuum in the vial.
    c. ensure sterile procedure.
    d. all of the above.

18. Epinephrine is an adrenergic drug that is classified as a

    a. depressant.   c. anticholinergic.
    b. stimulant.   d. antihistamine.

19. Drugs that are given to induce vomiting are classified as

    a. expectorants.   c. antipyretics.
    b. cathartics.   d. emetics.

20. The legislation that was passed in 1970 and, also, incorporates amendments to the Harrison Narcotic Act is known as the

    a. Pure Food and Drug Act.
    b. Durham-Humphrey Law.
    c. Controlled Substances Act of 1970.
    d. Federal Narcotic Control Law.

Section 5
Routine Laboratory Techniques

Unit 28 General Principles of Laboratory Operations

OBJECTIVES

Upon completion of this unit, the student should be able to

- State the general principles of laboratory operation.
- Identify various types of glassware used in laboratories.
- Explain how to properly clean glassware.
- Demonstrate the proper handling of reagents.

Some of the basic principles and rules of laboratory operations will be discussed in this unit. This is one area that requires absolute concentration and accuracy at all times and on all procedures. One way to ensure the accuracy of the laboratory work is to test the methods at least once a week.

PRINCIPLES

Some basic principles of laboratory operation are:

- The laboratory area should be maintained in a clean, neat, and well-stocked condition at all times.
- The working area should be free of clutter to provide adequate working space.
- Use only materials and solutions that have not become weakened or outdated. All equipment should be spotlessly clean.
- When working with caustic materials protect the working surface. Protect oneself with a laboratory coat or apron.
- Be sure that the proper methods of handling and cleaning glassware are known and used.

- Be extremely careful with Bunsen burners or alcohol burners as there are many flammable materials and solutions surrounding the laboratory area. Always turn them off when not in use.
- Dispose of staining solutions correctly. Pour them directly into the drain of the laboratory sink, not just into the sink.
- Know what to do immediately if a strong solution should be spilled on the skin.

    Acid: Rinse immediately with cold, running water. Neutralize the acid by applying an alkaline or base to the

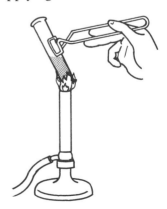

Fig. 28-1 Heating liquid in test tube over a Bunsen burner.

affected area as soon as the area has been thoroughly rinsed. Baking soda (soda bicarbonate) is an effective alkaline substance.

Alkali: Rinse immediately with cold, running water. Neutralize the alkali by applying a diluted acid to the affected area after it has been rinsed. Vinegar diluted with water is an effective acid solution.

• Always be familiar with the equipment, materials, and reagents that are being worked with.

• Do not attempt any laboratory tests that you have not been trained to do.

HANDLING GLASSWARE

Never use chipped or cracked glassware. Severe injuries such as lacerations or glass punctures may be sustained if damaged glassware is not discarded immediately.

Always clean glassware as soon as possible after use. If it cannot be cleaned immediately, put it in a soaking solution until it can be thoroughly cleaned. All glassware should be cleaned with hot, soapy water, rinsed completely, and if possible, dried in a hot air oven. If a hot air oven is not available, do *not* dry the glassware with cloth. Cloth leaves lint on glass. Invert the glassware on a rack and allow the air to dry it.

Glass slides should be cleaned with hot, soapy water, rinsed completely, and then soaked in a 95% alcohol. After the alcohol soak, they may be dried with a lint-free paper towel or special cleaning tissues which are used to clean slides. They are then stored in a dust free container such as a slide-storage box.

Pipettes and glass syringes that have contained blood should be soaked in a solution that dissolves blood. The barrel and plunger of the syringe are separated before being placed into any soaking solution. Blood-dissolving solutions can be purchased from a reliable chemical company; they are not as dangerous or as flammable as solutions which may be prepared in the medical office.

After the blood has been dissolved, the pipettes and syringes are washed with hot, soapy water, rinsed in clear water, and allowed to dry. This time-consuming procedure is not necessary if disposable pipettes and syringes are available.

Kinds of Glassware

A beaker is a wide-mouth container that is used for liquids. It has a pouring lip on one side of the upper edge of the beaker. Beakers may be Pyrex (a brand that is heatproof) or

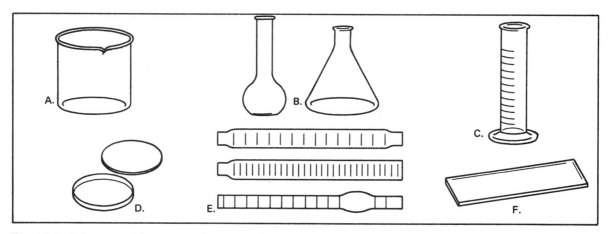

Fig. 28-2 Laboratory Glassware: A) beaker; B) flasks; C) graduated cylinder; D) Petri dish & cover; E) pipettes; F) slide.

simply glass. Before heating any glassware, check to be sure that it is flameproof. All Pyrex glassware is marked with a Pyrex symbol. Beakers are available in various sizes.

Flasks are containers that are wider at the bottom and smaller at the top with a neck similar to a bottle. They may or may not be Pyrex. Check before heating. Flasks may be stoppered with rubber or cork stoppers if necessary. Some flasks may be marked with graduated marks on the neck. These are called *volumetric flasks.*

Graduated cylinders are glass cylinders marked with volume lines that hold and measure liquids. They are available in various sizes.

Petri dishes are glass dishes, round and flat, with glass covers that are designed to hold culture media such as agar.

Microscope slides are flat, rectangular shaped glass plates that are used to prepare specimens to be viewed under the microscope. The specimen is put on the slide then fixed by one of several methods so that it will remain on the slide and be visible for observing.

Pipettes are long, narrow glass tubes that are graduated or marked with volume measurements. They are used to transfer liquids from one container or place to another. Some pipettes have bulbs that are used to draw the solution up into the pipette. Never attempt to suction solutions of any type into a pipette

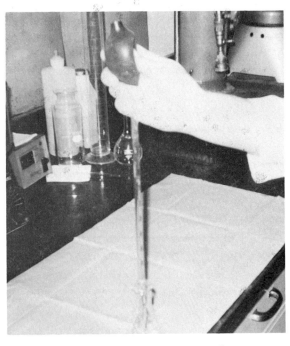

Fig. 28-3   Using a pipette to **transfer reagents.**

with the mouth. This is obviously a very dangerous practice since many of the reagents used in laboratories are very caustic and poisonous.

HANDLING REAGENTS

Always read the label on the bottle that is being handled. Be absolutely certain that the bottle is the correct one since the wrong reagent added to some substances can result in explosions and fires. Any unlabeled bottle should be destroyed immediately. Empty the

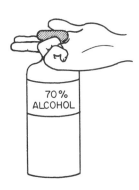

Fig. 28-4 Removing glass stopper from reagent bottle.

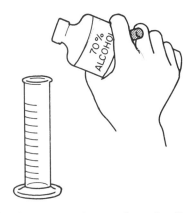

Fig. 28-5 Pouring reagent into graduated cylinder.

contents and discard the bottle. Do not attempt to identify a reagent by smelling its contents. The reagent may be poisonous and the fumes may damage the sensitive mucous membranes of the respiratory tract.

To open a reagent bottle with a glass stopper, grasp the glass stopper between the first and second fingers from the backside of the hand. Hold the stopper (see figure 28-5) while the reagent is being poured from the bottle. Do not lay the glass stopper down! If the reagent bottle has a screw top, remove it and lay it upside down on the countertop. Do not contaminate the inner area of the top. Always replace the reagent bottle's cap or stopper as soon as the solution has been removed from the bottle.

Never pour excess reagents back into the stock bottle. Pour a small amount into a smaller container and then measure the amount. More reagent can always be added but any excess reagent must be thrown away which is very expensive. Dry chemicals should be measured in the same manner. If reagents become contaminated, they are worse than useless to laboratory work. Contaminated reagents can cause laboratory results to be totally incorrect even though the procedure was executed accurately.

Mixing Reagents

When mixing any acid with water, always add the acid to the water. NEVER ADD THE WATER TO THE ACID. Adding water to some acids can result in powerful explosions.

Be certain that any solutions prepared in the laboratory are properly labeled. The solution is stored in a clean reagent bottle with a label identifying its contents and the date the solution was made. Be certain that the container storing the solution is absolutely clean. If the container is not clean the solution will be contaminated and laboratory tests will be inaccurate.

SUMMARY

Any procedure carried out in a laboratory must be done with the utmost care and knowledge. All principles relating to laboratory work must be observed at all times for the protection of the operator as well as for the absolute accuracy of the tests done. The accuracy of the laboratory equipment and supplies should be tested at least once a week. This can be done by running controlled tests on a normal person.

All rules, principles, and hazards must be known and observed at all times by everyone working in a laboratory setting.

SUGGESTED ACTIVITIES

- Arrange a visit to the laboratory of a nearby hospital. Observe the care and precision that is used in a laboratory setting.

- Invite a laboratory technician to speak to the class about routine laboratory care. Ask the technician to bring some of the most frequently used glassware. Question the technician about the methods of assuring accuracy in hospital laboratory tests.

REVIEW

A. Select the type of glassware from column II which applies to the description in column I.

I	**II**
1. _____ Any glassware that is flameproof.	a. slides
2. _____ Glass containers that are smaller at the top than the bottom.	b. pipettes
	c. beaker
3. _____ Straight-sided glass containers that are marked to indicate how much liquid it contains.	d. petri dishes
	e. flasks
4. _____ Straight-sided glass container that holds liquids and has a lip for pouring. Used for mixing reagents.	f. graduated cylinders
	g. Pyrex
5. _____ Round flat dishes that hold culture media and have covers.	
6. _____ Long, narrow tubes that are used to transfer liquids.	

B. Answer the following questions.

   1. List ten basic principles of laboratory operation.

   2. How should the following be cleaned?

       a. Glassware.

       b. Glass slides.

       c. Pipettes and syringes.

   3. What happens when reagents become contaminated?

   4. What should be done if acid is spilled on the skin?

5. What should be done if a strong alkali is spilled on the skin?

6. How should staining solutions be properly disposed of?

7. Why should a medical assistant *never* attempt to identify a reagent in an unlabeled bottle by smelling it?

8. Explain the proper method of opening a reagent bottle with a glass stopper.

9. Explain the proper method of opening a reagent bottle with a screw top.

10. How should reagents be measured when pouring them from a stock bottle?

11. When mixing any acid with water, always add the _____ to the _____. Why?

Unit 29 The Microscope

OBJECTIVES

After completing this unit, the student should be able to

- Correctly name the parts of the microscope.

- Demonstrate how to use the microscope.

In order to be able to function in the laboratory of a doctor's office, the medical assistant must be able to correctly use and care for a microscope.

Microscopes may either be monocular or binocular. A *monocular microscope* has only one eyepiece. Although the specimen will be viewed with only one eye, both eyes are kept open to avoid excessive eyestrain. A *binocular microscope* has two eyepieces. It takes a little more practice to be able to see through both eyepieces simultaneously.

PARTS OF THE MICROSCOPE

The *eyepiece* is the upper part of the tube, figure 29-1. Each eyepiece contains a lens that magnifies the object being viewed; it may be marked with 5X, 6X, or sometimes 10X. As mentioned before, there may be one (monocular) or two (binocular) eyepieces.

The *body tube* leads to the revolving nosepiece.

The *objectives* are small tubes attached to the nosepiece which revolves. There are

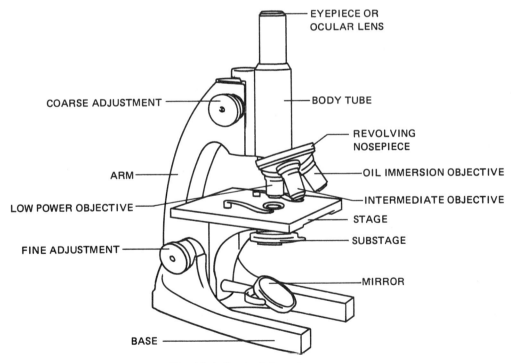

Fig. 29-1 Parts of the microscope.
(Courtesy of Bausch & Lomb Optical Company)

usually three objectives; each objective has different power. For example, the low power objective (which is the shortest one on the nosepiece) magnifies 10 times or 10X; the intermediate objective magnifies about forty times or 40X, and the high power objective (the longest one) magnifies about 100 times or 100X. The intermediate objective is used for high dry power. The high power objective is most often called the oil-immersion objective since it is used with oil-immersion technique.

The *stage* is the part that holds the slide under the objective. There are two clips, one on each side of the stage, that hold the slide in place. Located beneath the stage is a *substage* which holds a condenser that regulates the amount of light on the object under magnification. The condenser has a shutter or *diaphragm* that can shut out light or allow more light as needed. The substage may be raised or lowered to assist in focusing the slide.

The *arm* of the microscope supports the eyepiece. This is the part of the microscope that is held with the other hand underneath the base to support the microscope when it is necessary to move it.

The *base* is the part of the microscope that rests upon the table or work surface.

In addition to the parts mentioned already, there is a *coarse adjustment knob* and a *fine adjustment knob*.

A microscope must also have a light source such as a built-in lamp or a *mirror* for indirect lighting.

USE OF THE MICROSCOPE

Before using the microscope, the assistant must be sure that all mascara is removed from the eyelashes. Mascara gets oil and dirt on the ocular lens that is very hard to remove. To remove dust from the ocular lens, wipe it carefully with a special tissue that will not scratch the lens.

Place a slide with a hair on it between the clips on the stage. Focus the coarse adjustment until a wide shaft can be seen through the 10X or low power objective. After the outline of the hair can be seen, turn the fine adjustment knob until the edges of the hair can be seen very distinctly. The purpose of the fine adjustment is to bring detail into focus after the object has been found with the coarse adjustment.

If the hair cannot be brought into focus, check to be sure the hair is directly underneath the low power objective. Check the light source for adequate illumination. If the view is blurred, check the lens to be sure they are not dirty or smudged. If so, clean with the special tissue for microscope lens.

Do not raise the substage while looking through the eyepiece since this may result in forcing the lens of the objective through the slide, thus breaking the lens and/or the slide.

When using the oil-immersion objective, use the immersion oil sparingly and clean the objective lens carefully after use. Always use a cover slide with the oil-immersion objective. This protects the slide that is being examined. A clean slide can be used as a cover slide.

Always be aware of how close the objective lens is to the slide since damage to the microscope can occur if extreme care is not used. The objective used with oil-immersion technique will almost touch the slide but in actuality it will only touch the oil resting on the slide. That is the closest the objective should come to the slide.

If eyeglasses are worn, the microscope should be focused without the glasses as this will give a much clearer view. The microscope can be focused to compensate for visual defects except in the case of astigmatism.

Use of the microscope requires much patience and practice. The beginner should obtain this practice under the supervision of someone experienced in microscopy since the microscope is a very delicate and expensive instrument.

SUMMARY

The medical assistant must learn to use the microscope safely as well as learn the various parts of it. This experience should be gained under the supervision of someone experienced in microscopy.

SUGGESTED ACTIVITIES

- Draw a microscope and label the various parts.
- Under strict supervision in the school laboratory, arrange to use the microscope.
- Look at the following specimens under a microscope: Scraping from the inside of the mouth, saliva, a hair, a drop of urine, and scraping from the scalp.

REVIEW

A.   Label the parts of the microscope in figure 29-2.

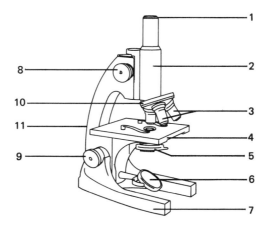

Fig. 29-2 **Parts of the microscope.**

1.   _____
2.   _____
3.   _____
4.   _____
5.   _____
6.   _____
7.   _____
8.   _____
9.   _____
10. _____
11. _____

Unit 30 Routine Urinalysis

OBJECTIVES

After studying this unit, the student should be able to

- State three types of examinations included in a routine urinalysis.
- List the tests that are included in each type of examination.
- Measure a specific gravity of urine.
- Prepare a urine specimen for a microscopic examination.

Most medical assistants will be required to do routine urinalysis exams. A routine urinalysis includes three types of examinations. They are a physical exam, a chemical exam, and a microscopic exam.

PHYSCIAL EXAMINATION OF URINE

The physical exam includes the general appearance of urine such as color, concentration, clarity, and odor. The exam also includes other tests such as specific gravity and pH. The color may range from colorless to straw color to dark yellow or even to amber or reddish brown.

The concentration is indicated by the intensity of the color. Generally pale urine is dilute while dark urine is concentrated. However, a color change may be caused by medication, dehydration, and the presence of abnormal substances in the urine. Very concentrated urine is noted on the urinalysis report.

The *clarity* of urine is noted. Urine is either clear, slightly cloudy, moderately cloudy, or very cloudy. The cloudiness found in some urines may be caused by large amounts of pus, bacteria, mucus, or phosphates and urates.

The *specific gravity* of urine must also be included in the physical exam. Specific gravity is the comparison of a given amount of urine to the same amount of water. The specific

gravity of water is 1. The specific gravity of normal urine ranges from 1.012 to 1.030.

Specific gravity is measured with a urinometer, figure 30-1. The urine is placed in the urinometer cylinder. The float is given a spin with the fingers so that it will not adher to the cylinder. When the float stops spinning, the specific gravity is read at eye level; the line of vision must be level with the lower line of the curve which crosses the scale of the float, figure 30-1. (The *meniscus* is the uneven line of the surface of the liquid.)

The degree of acidity or alkalinity of urine must also be measured; it is called *the pH* and

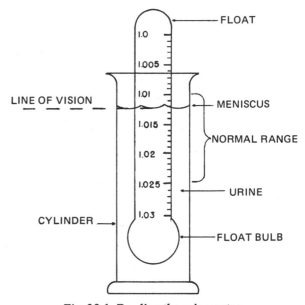

Fig. 30-1 Reading the urinometer.

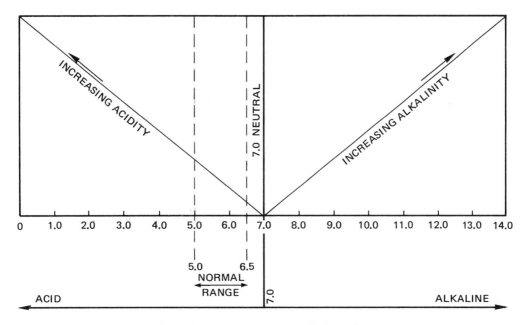

Fig. 30-2 Reaction or pH scale for urine.

ranges from 1 to 14. Determination of the pH of urine is called the *reaction*. The reaction is tested by dipping a strip of commercially prepared paper into the urine, waiting a prescribed amount of time and then comparing the color of the test strip to the color chart given. This will give a reading of the pH level. A reading below 7.0 is acid and above 7.0 is alkaline. A reading between 5.0 and 6.5 is considered within normal range.

CHEMICAL EXAMINATION

The chemical examination includes tests to determine:

- sugar (glucose, dextrose)
- albumin (protein)
- acetone (ketones)
- bilirubin
- urobilinogen
- porphyrins
- phenylketones (PKU)
- blood

These tests should be run on freshly voided urine. There are several methods of doing a chemical examination of urine. The safest, simplest methods that are most frequently used in physicians' offices will be given here. The testing equipment comes complete with everything necessary to run the test including clear, concise instructions.

To test the amount of glucose or sugar in the urine, either Diastix (test strips) or Clinitest tablets may be used. If the tablets are used, the medical assistant proceeds in the following manner.

- Place 5 drops of urine in a clean test tube.
- Rinse the dropper thoroughly.
- Add 10 drops of water to the urine in the tube.
- Drop 1 Clinitest tablet in the test tube. *Do not shake.*
- Observe the boiling action.
- *After* the boiling action stops, time for 15 seconds.
- Shake gently and compare with color chart.
- Record results.

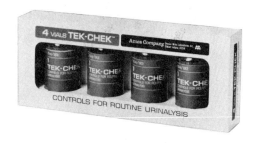

Fig. 30-3 Urinalysis control test.

Following are meanings of the colors obtained:

Color	Reading	Glucose percentage
Blue	Negative	0%
Green	Trace	1/4%
Green	+ (1 plus)	1/2%
Green	++ (2 plus)	3/4%
Brown	+++ (3 plus)	1%
Orange	++++ (4 plus)	2%

Note: The greens are different shades and should be compared against the color chart.

Another method to determine the presence of glucose in the urine is to use the test strip method. Combistix (Ames) are test strips that measure the pH, glucose, and protein in urine with one test procedure. The strip is dipped into urine and then read or compared with the color chart on the bottle at specified times in good lighting. Keto-Diastix reagent strips measure glucose and ketones in urine.

Today, commercially prepared test strips are available for many different types of urine testing. For example, packaged units are available for running a *control test* for routine urinalysis; this is a method of checking testing techniques and materials for accuracy.

Other commercially-prepared testing products are available such as reagent strips and tablets for testing for protein, blood, ketones, bilirubin, urobilinogen, pH, and phenylketones.

MICROSCOPIC EXAMINATION

For a microscopic examination, the urine specimen is first stirred or shaken to prevent

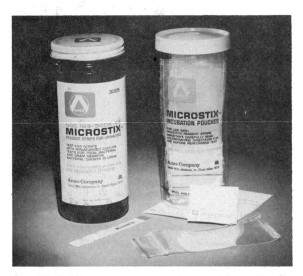

Fig. 30-4 Microstix reagent strips used in testing for nitrate with culture tests for bacterial counts.

settlement of sediment. A sample of 10 cc of the urine is placed in a centrifuge tube. The sample is centrifuged for 5 minutes at 1,500 revolutions per minute. All of the sample is then poured out of the centrifuge tube, except for a few remaining drops and the sediment in the bottom of the tube.

The few remaining drops are mixed thoroughly with the sediment. Transfer a drop of the mixture to a slide with a capillary pipette. Cover the drop with a cover glass or slide and place it on the stage of the microscope.

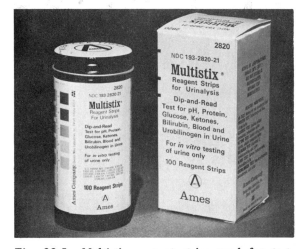

Fig. 30-5 Multistix reagent strips used for testing pH, protein, glucose, ketones, bilirubin, blood and urobilinogen.

CRYSTALS FOUND IN ACID URINE 400 X

Uric acid | Amorphous urates and uric acid crystals | Hippuric acid | Calcium oxalate | Tyrosine needles Leucine spheroids Cholesterin plates

CRYSTALS FOUND IN ALKALINE URINE 400 X

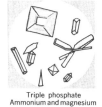 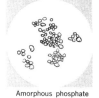 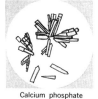 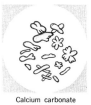 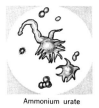

Triple phosphate Ammonium and magnesium | Triple phosphate going in solution | Amorphous phosphate | Calcium phosphate | Calcium carbonate | Ammonium urate

SULFA CRYSTALS

Sulfanilamide | Sulfathiazole | Sulfadiazine | Sulfapyridine

CELLS FOUND IN URINE

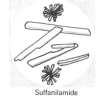 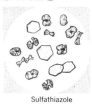 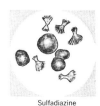 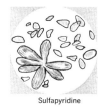 

RBC and WBC | Renal epithelium | Caudate cells of Renal Pelvis | Urethral and bladder epithelium | Vaginal epithelium | Yeast and bacteria

CASTS AND ARTIFACTS FOUND IN URINE 400 X

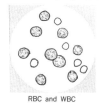 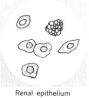 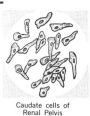 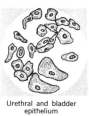 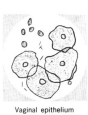 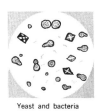

Granular casts fine and coarse | Hyaline cast | Leukocyte cast | Epithelial cast | Waxy cast | Blood cast

 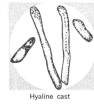 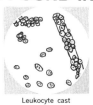 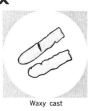 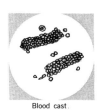

Cylindroids | Mucous thread | Spermatozoa | Trichomonas vaginalis | Cloth fibers and bubbles

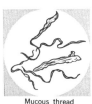 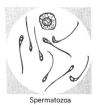 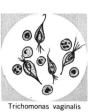 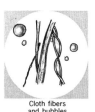 

Fig. 30-6 Crystals, cells, and casts found in urine sediment.

PHYSICAL EXAMINATION:

Appearance *Clear, Straw-colored*

pH *4.5 to 7.5*   Specific Gravity *1.010 to 1.025*

CHEMICAL ANALYSIS:

Albumin (protein) *None to trace*   Urobilinogen *NEG.*

Sugar (glucose, dextrose) *None*   Porphyrins *NEG.*

Ketones (acetone) *None*   PKU *NEG.*

Bilirubin *None*   Occult Blood *NEG.*

MICROSCOPIC EXAMINATION:

Cells: Epithelial *few*

WBC's *0 to 4*

RBC's *few to occasional*

Casts: Hyaline *NEG.*

Epithelial *NEG.*

Blood *NEG.*

Crystals: *few*

Other: *NEG.*

Fig. 30-7 Table of normal values for a routine urinalysis.

Using the low power objective, examine the slide for casts and epithelial cells. A dark field is necessary to see if casts are present. Epithelial cells are counted or reported as few, moderate, or many. Casts are reported in the same manner.

Both normal and abnormal crystals will be found with the high power objective and should be identified. Uric acid crystals, calcium oxalates, amorphous urates, phosphates, and ammonium biurate crystals may be found in normal urine. Leucine, tyrosine, cystine, and cholesterol crystals may be found in abnormal urine.

Other materials sometimes noted in urine on microscopic examinations are protozoa called trichomonas vaginalis, yeast cells, and mold fungi. All of these materials as well as the crystals must be recognized by the med-ical assistant who is expected to do urine examinations.

SUMMARY

A urinalysis includes a physical examination, a chemical examination, and a microscopic examination. The physical examination consists of a determination of color, clarity, concentration, odor, pH, and specific gravity of the specimen.

A chemical examination consists of the determination of sugar or glucose content, albumin, acetone, and sometimes other substances such as urobilinogen, bilirubin, blood, porphyrins, or phenylketones.

A microscopic examination includes a determination of cells, casts, crystals, or other materials that may be found in urine.

SUGGESTED ACTIVITIES

- Observe slides of the following materials found in the urine and learn to identify them.

    (1) epithelial cells

    (2) casts (hyaline, epithelial, and blood)

    (3) crystals found in both acid and alkaline urine

    (4) protozoa, yeast, and fungi cells sometimes found in urine

- Do a routine urinalysis, using your own urine as the specimen.

REVIEW

Briefly answer the following questions.

1. Name the three examinations included in a routine urinalysis.

2. Name six factors determined by the physical examination of urine.

3. a. What is the determination of the pH of urine called?

    b. How is it tested?

4. Describe how specific gravity is measured.

5. Name five tests included in the chemical examination of urine.

6. Explain the procedure for preparing a urine specimen for microscopic examination.

7. What power objective on the microscope is used to find epithelial cells and casts?

8. What power objective is used to determine the presence of crystals?

9. List four types of crystals that may be found in *abnormal* urine.

10. List five types of crystals that may be found in *normal* urine.

Unit 31 Hematology

OBJECTIVES

After completing the unit, the student should be able to

- State the normal values for hematocrit, hemoglobin, erythrocytes, and leukocytes.
- Count the erythrocytes in a blood sample.
- Count the leukocytes in a blood sample.
- Explain how to do a hemoglobin estimation.

Hematology is the study of the blood and its components. The hematology studies that are done in the physician's office are very limited and most are rough estimates rather than the precise results obtained in a hematology laboratory. Even so, the assistant must be as careful and as accurate as she can possibly be in all laboratory work.

ERYTHROCYTE COUNT

Erythrocytes or red blood cells derive their red color from *hemoglobin* which is an iron-carrying protein. The normal RBC count for men is 4½ million to 5½ million; for women it is 4 to 5 million.

Blood for the erythrocyte count is obtained from a finger puncture using a RBC pipette. The blood is drawn into the pipette to the 0.5 mark *exactly*. Excess blood on the outside of the pipette is wiped away. (All RBC pipettes are structured so that blood drawn to the 0.5 point and then diluted to the

101 point will result in a dilution of 1 : 200.) Draw RBC diluting fluid (Hayem's solution or 0.85% NaCl) into the pipette to the 101 point. Take great care that the blood in the pipette does not enter the stock diluting fluid. Using a figure eight motion, rotate the pipette for three minutes. Do *NOT* shake the pipette along its axis. After three minutes, discard 2 to 4 drops of the dilute blood from the pipette.

Drop a large drop from the pipette onto the chamber platform that has been properly covered with a clean cover slip. The drop should cover the ruled area but not the moat on the sides. The cover slip should not be moved after charging the chamber and there should be no air bubbles. After about two minutes, place the chamber on the microscope

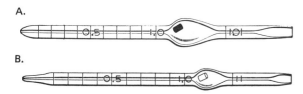

Fig. 31-1 Pipettes. (A) Red blood cell diluting pipette. (B) White blood cell diluting pipette.

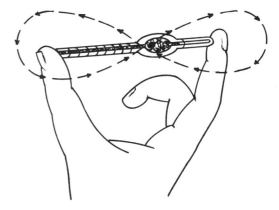

Fig. 31-2 Figure eight motion for mixing diluting solution with blood.

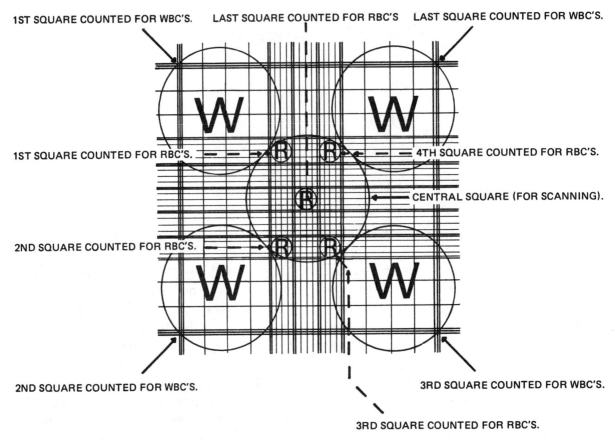

1ST SQUARE COUNTED FOR WBC'S.   LAST SQUARE COUNTED FOR RBC'S   LAST SQUARE COUNTED FOR WBC'S.

1ST SQUARE COUNTED FOR RBC'S.   4TH SQUARE COUNTED FOR RBC'S.

CENTRAL SQUARE (FOR SCANNING).

2ND SQUARE COUNTED FOR RBC'S.

2ND SQUARE COUNTED FOR WBC'S.   3RD SQUARE COUNTED FOR WBC'S.

3RD SQUARE COUNTED FOR RBC'S.

Fig. 31-3 Counting chamber field for RBC's and WBC's.

stage very carefully. Scan the central ruled area to see if the cells are distributed fairly equally. Use the low power objective for scanning. If the cells are equally distributed, switch to high power after moving the chamber so that the upper left secondary square is centered in the field of vision.

After adjusting the lighting and focus, count all the RBC's in the four corner squares and in the central square. Total all cells counted.

Find the number of RBC's by multiplying the total cells counted by 5, then by 10, then by 200, to find the number of cells per cubic millimeter, (total cells counted x5x10 x200). Or simply multiply the cells counted by 10,000, (5x10x200=10,000). The resulting number should give the number of RBC's per cubic millimeter.

LEUKOCYTE COUNT

The leukocyte count is the counting of white blood cells. WBC's fight bacteria and infection in the body. *Phagocytosis* is the process of white blood cells combating infection and forming pus. The normal WBC count is from 5,000 to 10,000 in both males and females. The average normal is around 7,500.

WBC pipettes are made so that blood drawn to the 0. 5 point and then diluted to the 11 mark will be a 1:20 solution, regardless of the size of the pipette. The procedure for a WBC count is basically the same as for a RBC count.

Using a WBC pipette and WBC diluting fluid (Turck's solution) collect from a drop of blood the correct amount in the WBC pipette (to the 0. 5 point). Dilute to the 11 mark with

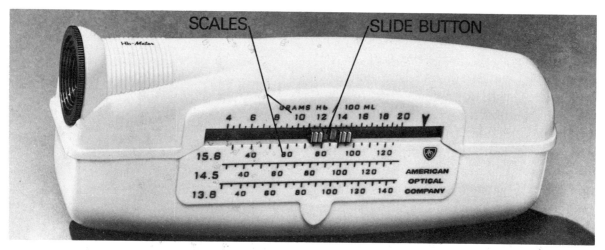

Fig. 31-4 Hemoglobinometer.
(Courtesy of American Optical Corp.)

WBC diluting solution. Discard two to four drops and then charge the counting chamber with a drop of the solution. Focus the chamber under low power objective and check for even distribution of the white cells. Still using low power, count the cells in the four primary squares. To calculate the total number of WBC's divide the total by 4 then multiply by 10, then by 20, (total ÷ 4x10x20). Or simply multiply the total number of cells in the four large squares by 50. The result is the number of white cells per cubic millimeter.

HEMOGLOBIN ESTIMATION

A hemoglobinometer is frequently used to estimate the hemoglobin or amount of iron-carrying protein in the blood.

The blood used for the measurement of hemoglobin can be taken from a finger puncture. A drop of blood taken from the total amount drawn from a venipuncture for several tests may also be used. If the blood is from a finger puncture, the drop can be placed directly onto the chamber surface. The cover slip is slightly offset when held in the clip so that the chamber surface is exposed to receive the blood.

The blood is then hemolyzed by agitating the blood with a hemolysis applicator included

in the apparatus. Whole blood has a cloudy appearance. Hemolysis breaks down the cell wall membranes which results in a transparent appearance of the hemolyzed blood. This process can be observed visually. The hemolysis process takes about 45 seconds to complete the change from cloudy to clear.

The offset chamber is pushed completely into the clip after hemolysis is completed. The

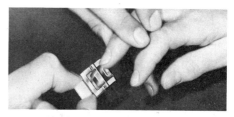
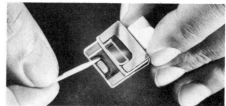
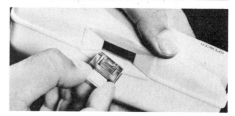

Fig. 31-5 Changing the chamber for the hemoglobinometer.

clipped chamber is then inserted into the slot on the left side of the hemoglobinometer. The instrument is placed to the eye with the left hand so that the left thumb can operate the light switch on the bottom of the instrument. When the light button is switched on, a split green field is visible. The right hand manipulates the slide button on the right side of the instrument until there is no difference in the light field. The split field should disappear completely. Take note of the position of the right-hand slide button. There are four scales present on the instrument. The most frequently used scale will be the top one which reads grams of hemoglobin per 100 milliliters.

The normal hemoglobin count for men ranges from 14 to 18 Gm/100 ml and for women the range is from 12 to 16 Gm/100 ml.

DIFFERENTIAL COUNT

The differential count will be discussed briefly but the procedure will not be given here as this is a very difficult technique to do correctly and requires much instruction and practice to become proficient. Most physicians prefer having the differential count done by an experienced technician in a well-equipped laboratory.

The differential count is the count of the various types of white blood cells. These different kinds of WBC are identified by observing specially stained slides under the oil-objective lens of the microscope.

Some normal mature leukocytes are:

- Polymorphonuclear cells. The nucleus has several lobes and the cytoplasm is granulated. After staining, they are further classified as neutrophils, eosinophils, or basophils.

- Mononuclear cells. The nucleus is usually round and well centered. There are two types of mononuclear cells which are classified after staining as lymphoctyes or monocytes.

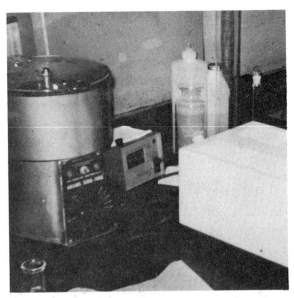

Fig. 31-6 Centrifuges used in hematocrit determinations.

Platelets may also be observed in a differential count although a special procedure is done for a platelet count. Platelets are thrombocytes or blood-clotting cells.

HEMATOCRIT

To determine the volume of packed red blood cells, a test called the *hematocrit* is done. Special apparatus is necessary to do a hematocrit. A centrifuge is required as well as a Wintrobe tube or hematocrit tube. Only venous blood can be used.

Venous blood is obtained from a venipuncture and is oxalated. The hematocrit tube is filled to the 0 (zero) point and placed in the centrifuge for 40 minutes at 3000 rpm's (revolutions per minute).

The reading is obtained from the right side of the scale after centrifuging is completed. The number of packed red cells is read and multiplied by 10 to give the number of packed red cells per 100 milliliters of blood.

The normal hematocrit for men is 43 to 59% or vol/100 ml and 40 to 47% or vol/100 ml for women.

SUMMARY

The hematology determinations most often done in the doctor's office are the erythrocyte count, the leukocyte count, the hemoglobin determination, and the hematocrit. Other tests such as the differential count or the platelet count are done in hematology labs by experienced technicians. However, the assistant should know what they are.

SUGGESTED ACTIVITIES

- Make arrangements to visit a hematology laboratory and observe experienced technicians performing hematology studies.

- Practice the hemoglobin determination and the hematocrit in the school laboratory.

- Prepare the slides and, under supervision, do an erythrocyte count and a leukocyte count.

- Locate a color plate of leukocytes and identify the various types of leukocytes on a commercially prepared, differential count slide.

REVIEW

A. Fill in the blanks with the correct word or words.

    1. Red blood cells are called _____ .

    2. White blood cells are called _____ .

    3. Red blood cells get their color from _____.

    4. A(n) _____ pipette is used to do a red blood count.

    5. A(n) _____ pipette is used to do a white blood count.

    6. A _____ is the apparatus used to make a hemoglobin determination.

B. Answer the following questions.

    1. What two pieces of laboratory equipment are necessary in order to do a hematocrit?

    2. What objective is used to view a stained slide for a differential count?

    3. Other than leukocytes, what can be seen on a differential count?

    4. What is the diluting fluid used for a WBC count?

5. What is the diluting fluid used for a RBC count?

6. Once the RBC's have been counted, what calculations do you use?

7. Once the WBC's have been counted, what calculations do you use?

C. Complete the following.
   1. Give the normal values for the following determinations.

      a. Hematocrit: women _____
                              men _____

      b. WBC's: men or women _____

      c. Hemoglobin: women _____
                              men _____

      d. RBC's: women _____
                              men _____

   2. The RBC pipette is filled to the _____ point with blood and then to the _____ point with _____. This results in a dilution ratio of _____.

   3. The WBC pipette is filled to the _____ point with blood and then to the _____ point with _____. This results in a dilution ratio of _____.

Unit 32 Blood Chemistry Determinations

OBJECTIVES

After completing this unit, the student should be able to

- State the normal blood sugar and blood urea nitrogen.
- Describe how to perform blood chemistry tests using reagent strips.
- Explain the use of a photometer.

Some blood chemistry determinations are simple enough to be done in the physician's office by the medical assistant by using reagent strips. Some offices also have an apparatus known as a blood analyzer or photometer; it simplifies and increases the number of blood chemistry tests that can be done. A blood sugar and a blood urea nitrogen test are two blood chemistry determinations which may be done in the office.

BLOOD SUGAR

The blood used for a blood sugar determination can be obtained from a finger puncture unless venous blood is already available. The testing is usually done with a reagent strip. Be sure the correct side of the strip is used.

Freely apply a large drop of capillary (or venous) blood to the test strip. Cover the entire testing area. Time the waiting period for exactly 60 seconds. Use a watch or clock with a second hand. Using a spray bottle, wash the blood off the strip with a short stream of water. Read the strip immediately, using the color chart on the test strip label. The reading will be the blood sugar determination.

Only whole blood is used for this test. The *timing must be absolutely accurate* in order to obtain correct results. This test for blood sugar, as with any other laboratory technique, requires practice until the medical assistant becomes proficient.

For greater accuracy, an instrument may be used with reagent strips, see figure 32-2.

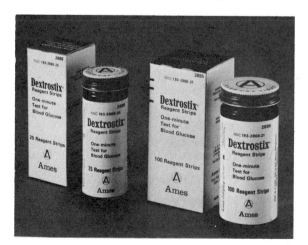

Fig. 32-1 **Reagent strips used for blood glucose readings.**

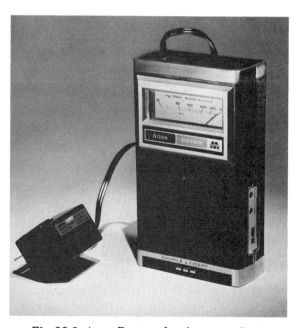

Fig. 32-2 **Ames Eyetone for glucose readings.**

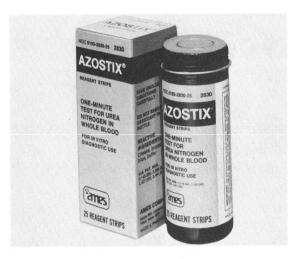

Fig. 32-3 Reagent strips for BUN test.

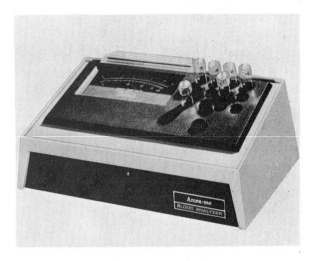

Fig. 32-4 A blood analyzer or photometer.

The procedure is the same except that instead of comparing the strip to the color chart on the label of the bottle, the strip is inserted into the instrument's strip guide. The lid is then pressed firmly in the center and observation of the meter needle is recorded. The meter reading ranges from 10 milligrams per 100 milliliters to 400 mg/100 ml. The normal blood sugar range in a fasting state is from 60 to 120 mg/100 ml of blood.

BLOOD UREA NITROGEN

A blood urea nitrogen determination (BUN) may be made by using specific reagent test strips. The instructions are on the bottle of test strips and are simple and easy to follow.

Capillary blood is used to saturate the test strip. The normal BUN ranges from 10 to 20 mg/100 ml of blood.

PHOTOMETERS

A photometer or blood analyzer is an instrument designed for blood chemistry analysis, figure 32-4. It is relatively easy to use and comes equipped with complete operating instructions. The photometer is an integrated system that uses reagent kits to do serum tests on albumin, bilirubin, BUN, cholesterol, creatinine, hemoglobin, and many other tests.

SUMMARY

Blood chemistries consist of various tests run on blood samples to determine the blood sugar content, the blood urea nitrogen (BUN), the cholesterol, bilirubin, and many other blood elements.

In the doctor's office the blood chemistries are usually restricted to blood sugar or blood urea nitrogen determinations since the equipment and the skills necessary for most of the other chemistries are not available in the physician's office.

However, the availability of the newer photometers and blood analyzers have made it possible for more screening tests to be done in the doctor's office.

SUGGESTED ACTIVITIES

- Make arrangements to visit a physician's office to see a photometer or blood analyzer in operation.
- Practice doing blood sugar analysis and BUN's on classmates.

REVIEW

Select the answer that best completes each statement.

1. Blood obtained from a finger puncture is known as

   a. capillary blood.   c. arterial blood.
   b. venous blood.   d. diluted blood.

2. Blood used for a blood sugar determination can be quickly obtained from

   a. plasma.   c. whole blood.
   b. packed cells.   d. none of these.

3. The special apparatus used to determine a blood sugar reading using a reagent test strip is the

   a. photometer.   c. blood analyzer.
   b. eyetone.   d. colorimeter.

4. The normal BUN ranges from

   a. 60 to 120 mg/100 ml blood.
   b. 10 to 20 mg/100 ml blood.
   c. 10 mg to 400 mg/100 ml blood.
   d. none of the above.

5. A photometer or blood analyzer can analyze blood for

   a. blood sugar determinations.   c. hemoglobin.
   b. blood urea nitrogen.   d. all of these.

Unit 33 Bacteriology

OBJECTIVES

After completing this unit, the student should be able to

- Take a bacteriological smear and prepare it for staining.
- Stain a bacteriological smear.
- Differentiate between Gram-negative and Gram-positive reactions.
- Examine the stained slide microscopically.

Bacteriologic smears are prepared, usually by staining, to determine the presence or absence of bacteria from various areas of the body. Smears may be taken from the mouth, ear, nose, throat, eyes, skin surface, vagina, or any wound. If a bacteriologic smear indicates the presence of bacteria, the stained slide can often help identify the specific bacteria.

MAKING THE SMEAR

The physician, or the assistant if the physician wishes, may make the smear. The procedure for making a smear is relatively simple but important, as treatment of the patient may depend on the result.

- A sterile applicator or swab is introduced into the body area from which the smear is to be taken. Exudate (drainage) or a sample from the surface of the area is transferred to the applicator.
- Holding a clean glass slide between the thumb and forefinger of the left hand, the specimen is transferred from the applicator to the glass slide. To do this, the applicator must be rolled across the surface of the slide centered on the middle

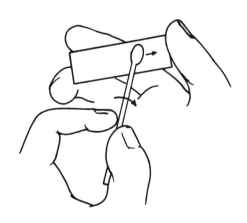

Fig. 33-1 Smearing the slide.

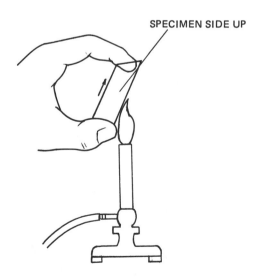

Fig. 33-2 Fixing the smear by flaming.

of the slide, figure 33-1. The applicator is *NOT* rubbed back and forth across the slide as this can cause damage to the bacteria and its grouping, making identification difficult.

- After transferring the specimen to the slide, the surface of the slide is allowed to dry at room temperature. The smear is then fixed by flaming; this is done to prevent the specimen from being washed away when it is being stained.

- To fix or flame the slide, hold it securely between the thumb and forefinger, specimen side up. Slowly pass it over a bunsen burner so that the flame barely touches the underside of the slide, figure 33-2. Repeat this procedure two or three times. The slide should not become too hot to handle or the elements to be identified will be destroyed. When flaming is completed, place the slide on a staining rack.

STAINING THE SLIDE

In order to make the fixed bacteria visible for study and identification, a staining process is used. The most often used staining process is the Gram stain. The bacteria that retain the violet-colored stain are *Gram-positive* bacteria. The bacteria that do not retain the stain are *Gram-negative* bacteria. Staining with the Gram stain is known as the Gram stain technique.

- The flamed slide is placed on the staining rack. The rack should be directly over the drain unless there is a catch tray to prevent staining of the counter top. This is truly a difficult stain to remove from clothing, hands, or other articles and should be handled very carefully.

- The fixed slide is covered with crystal or gentian violet and allowed to remain for 60 seconds. After one minute, pour water from a beaker onto the slide and tilt it so that the excess water and stain can run off. Using Gram's iodine, cover the slide again. Pour off by tilting the slide. Cover again with Gram's iodine and leave for 60 seconds. Wash with water from beaker.

- Decolorize with 95% ethyl alcohol (or acetone) by holding the slide at one end and covering it with the decolorizer, tilting the slide to allow the decolorizer to run off, covering again, tilting and observing the decolorizer as it runs off the slide. The decolorizing process should only take a very few seconds and great care must be taken not to decolorize excessively. As soon as the decolorizer runs off the slide without any purple color, stop decolorizing. Wash with water immediately.

- Counterstain by covering the slide with safranin solution or dilute fuchsin. Pour the counterstain off the slide immediately. Flood with water. Wipe excess solution from the back of the slide and allow the stained surface to air dry.

After the slide has dried, the stain is fairly permanent. However, since these stained slides are observed under the oil-immersion objective, a cover glass is recommended to preserve the stain which can be damaged by the oil and the oil remover. Using a cover glass will preserve the slide for an indefinite amount of time and viewings.

MICROSCOPIC EXAMINATION

Now that the slide has been stained, it is ready for analysis. The oil-immersion objective is used for the microscopic examination.

Note the formation or the groupings of the bacteria. Remember, cocci are found in clusters or special groupings. Staphylococci are in grapelike clusters, diplococci are in pairs, and streptococci are in chains.

How are they shaped? Do they have capsulated coverings? Review unit 7 for microbial identification.

Any bacteria that shows a purple stain is called Gram-positive bacteria and the bacteria that shows a red stain is Gram-negative bacteria. Smears may contain different kinds of bacteria and will be classified as either Gram-negative or Gram-positive.

Some Gram-negative microorganisms are: the gonococci that cause gonorrhea; the typhoid bacilli that cause typhoid fever and is known as Salmonella typhosa; and the Bordetella pertussis that causes whooping cough. Examples of organisms that are Gram-positive are: the tubercle bacillus that causes tuberculosis; the streptococci; and the staphylococci. Of course there are many more but these are a few examples.

PRECAUTIONS

While doing microbiological studies, the assistant must remember at all times that she is dealing with live organisms. The only protection from the disease is her technique in handling these organisms.

All pathogenic organisms are considered dangerous and communicable. The assistant is handling contaminated materials and must be aware of this at all times. Proper handwashing and disposal of contaminated materials *must* be done.

After checking the stained slide, the assistant may make her own observations about the contents of the slide but the actual determination of what kind of organisms the slide contains is made only by the physician. Note: It is not in the realm of the assistant's duties to actually decide what the organism is or to say that the patient has a certain condition or disease based upon her observations. Only the physician's experience and training are adequate for these conclusions.

SUMMARY

The doctor or the medical assistant may make a smear from which a slide is prepared. The assistant can only do this with the physician's permission.

The smear is then fixed or flamed, and stained. The Gram staining technique indicates whether bacteria is Gram-positive or Gram-negative by showing which bacteria retain the Gram stain.

The stained slide is then viewed under the microscope using the oil-immersion objective. If the slide is to be preserved, a cover glass should be applied before the microscopic examination. The doctor examines the slide and makes the actual analysis but the assistant should be able to identify the different types of bacteria.

Proper technique must be observed at all times.

SUGGESTED ACTIVITIES

- View some stained slides and identify the microorganisms present. Identify the Gram-positive and the Gram-negative organisms.

- Prepare a slide for staining. Use a smear from the inside of the cheek.

- Practice staining techniques and making a smear. Take a smear from the throat or from any wound or lesion that might be present.

REVIEW

A. Identify the types of organisms found in the illustration on page 195.

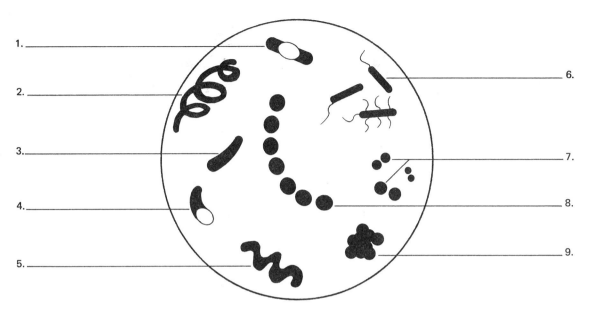

1.
2.
3.
4.
5.
6.
7.
8.
9.

Microbacteria Identification

B. Select the answer that best completes the following statements.

   1. A smear may be obtained by taking a sample specimen from various body areas by using a

   a. lancet.   c. cotton ball.
   b. cotton applicator.   d. sterile sponge.

   2. Heating the specimen on the slide is called

   a. fixing the slide.
   b. staining the slide.
   c. counterstaining the slide.
   d. smearing the slide.

   3. The process that determines whether bacteria is Gram-positive or Gram-negative is called

   a. staining.   c. Gram-staining.
   b. fixing.   d. decolorizing.

   4. If purple staining dye washes off the bacteria and leaves it red instead of purple, the bacteria is

   a. Gram-positive.   c. nonstainable.
   b. Gram-negative.   d. unidentifiable.

   5. Gram stain is easily removed by using

   a. water.   c. safranin.
   b. acetone.   d. none of these.

Self-Evaluation Test 5

Select the answers that best complete the following statements.

1. The antidote that should be applied immediately after rinsing acid from the skin is

   a. vinegar.
   b. alcohol.
   c. soda bicarbonate.
   d. soap and water.

2. Glass slides used in the laboratory are washed, rinsed, and soaked in

   a. 70% alcohol.
   b. 95% alcohol.
   c. zephiren.
   d. phenol.

3. Laboratory glassware that bears the small inscription, *Pyrex,* is

   a. heatproof.
   b. unbreakable.
   c. disposable.
   d. all of these.

4. Graduated glass tubes that are used to transfer liquids from one container or one place to another are

   a. volumetric cylinders.
   b. pipettes.
   c. flasks.
   d. beakers.

5. The parts of the microscope that are attached to the nosepiece are the

   a. eyepieces.
   b. objectives.
   c. substage.
   d. none of these.

6. A cover slide is used when using the oil-immersion objective to

   a. protect the lens of the objective.
   b. magnify the contents of the slide.
   c. prevent distortion of the view through the oil.
   d. protect the slide that is being examined.

7. The specific gravity of normal urine ranges from

   a. 1.012 to 1.030.
   b. 6.0 to 6.5.
   c. 1.01 to 1.10.
   d. none of these.

8. Before a microscopic examination of urine can be run, the urine must be

   a. heated to 48.9°C (120°F)
   b. centrifuged.
   c. filtered.
   d. stirred thoroughly.

9. Crystals found in the urine during a microscopic examination indicate a

   a. normal condition.
   b. abnormal condition.
   c. disease or injury.
   d. need to distinguish between normal and abnormal crystals.

10. The study of blood and its components is known as

    a. bacteriology.
    b. hematology.
    c. blood chemistry determinations.
    d. all of the above.

11. The normal erythrocyte count (per cubic millimeter) for women is

    a. 4 to 5 million.   c. 5,000 to 10,000.
    b. 4½ to 5½ million.   d. none of these.

12. The process of hemolysis that is done before measuring hemoglobin is done to

    a. coagulate the blood.
    b. break down the cell wall membranes.
    c. cause a cloudy appearance to occur in the blood.
    d. all of the above.

13. The normal hemoglobin count for men is

    a. 12 to 16 Gm/100 ml.   c. 14 to 18 Gm/100 ml.
    b. 12 to 16 Gm/1000 mm.   d. 14 to 18 Gm/1000 mm.

14. The normal leukocyte count for men and women is

    a. 4 to 5 million.   c. 12,000 to 15,000.
    b. 4½ to 5½ million.   d. 5,000 to 10,000.

15. In order to do a hematocrit, the blood used for testing must be

    a. oxalated arterial blood.
    b. oxalated venous blood.
    c. blood obtained from a finger puncture.
    d. nonoxalated blood.

16. All of the following tests may be done in a physician's office during hematological determinations except for the

    a. erythrocyte count.   c. hemoglobin count.
    b. leukocyte count.   d. differential count.

17. The *two* blood chemistries that might be run in a doctor's office without a photometer would be the

    a. blood urea nitrogen.   c. platelet count.
    b. cholesterol count.   d. blood sugar determinations.

18. Staining slides for microscopic examination is done in order to

    a. fix organisms on a slide so they won't wash off.
    b. fix organisms on a slide so they can't contaminate the medical assistant.
    c. determine the presence or absence of bacteria.
    d. all of the above.

19. The bacteria that retains the violet-colored stain during the staining process is

    a. Gram-positive bacteria.   c. pathogenic bacteria.
    b. Gram-negative bacteria.   d. counterstained bacteria.

20. The main thing that stands between the medical assistant and disease when she is working with bacteriological studies is

    a. the flaming process that fixes the slide.
    b. knowing if the bacteria are of the spore-forming type before handling the slides.
    c. ensuring that her vaccinations are all kept up to date.
    d. her own technique in handling these microorganisms.

Section 6
Other Diagnostic Procedures

Unit 34 Hospital Departments and Diagnostic Tests

OBJECTIVES

After completing this unit, the student should be able to

- Indicate the functions of specific departments where diagnostic procedures are performed.
- Classify a given list of diagnostic tests.

In addition to the diagnostic tests that have been discussed in previous units, there are many tests and procedures that cannot be done in the doctor's office. These procedures require expensive, complicated equipment and specially trained people to administer the tests and read the results.

CLINICAL LABORATORY

The *clinical laboratory* is a highly specialized department found in hospitals and clinics. Its function is to carry out technical laboratory tests. Special analysis are done on blood, urine, sputum, tissue fluids, feces, and other secretions or fluids of the body. The

physician must order the desired test; the assistant makes the arrangements to have those tests carried out. Some tests require special preparation by the patient. The assistant must be sure the patient has all the instructions necessary before presenting himself for the tests.

PATHOLOGY

Pathology is the study of the nature of disease and its cause. Examination of the body tissues is an important part of this study. Clinical pathology is a specialty area that deals

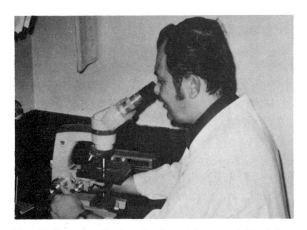

Fig. 34-1 A medical technologist has special training in the examination of specimens.

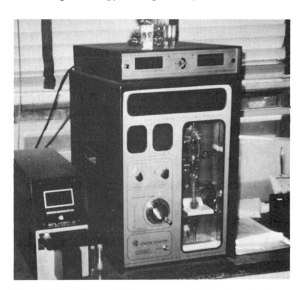

Fig. 34-2 Hemoglobinometer and Photometer in a clinical lab.

with tissue *morphology* (the study of structure and form); these studies determine whether tissues are normal or abnormal. If abnormal, pathology determines what the abnormality is. An example of the function of pathology is the study of biopsies. A *biopsy* is the excision of a small piece of body tissue for study purposes. For example, bone marrow or lymphatic tissue may be examined in suspected leukemia. Pathology may determine whether or not tissues are healthy. If tissues are not healthy, pathology may determine, by microscopic study, the type of illness present in the tissues.

NUCLEAR MEDICINE

Nuclear medicine is a highly specialized area where diagnostic studies are made and therapeutic treatments are given. Nuclear medicine is concerned with ionizing radiation and the use of radioisotopes on the body. One diagnostic procedure follows the progress of special radioisotopes in the body to determine thyroid efficiency. The process of the radioisotopes is followed carefully and is recorded on a graph by a special scanner. The results can establish a thyroid deficiency. The physician who requests the tests and gets the results can then order medication to compensate for deficiency.

DIAGNOSTIC TESTS

The medical assistant should be familiar with all of the diagnostic tests that the physician might order on a patient. The following are some common diagnostic tests.

Liver Function Tests

> Alkaline phosphatase determination
> Bilirubin tolerance
> Blood thrombin determination
> Galactose tolerance test
> Serum transaminase (SGOT and SGPT)
> Thymol turbidity
> Serum cholesterol

Renal Function Tests

> Glomerular Function
> > Glomerular filtration rate
> > PAH clearance
> > Urea clearance
> Renal Blood Flow
> > Blood urea clearance
> > Hippuric acid clearance
> Renal Tubular Function
> > Concentration tests
> > Phenol red excretion (PSP)
> > Methylene blue excretion

GI Tract Tests

> Gastric acid determination
> Gastric pH
> Gastric emptying time

Endocrine System Tests

> Basal Metabolic Rate (BMR)
> Radioactive iodine uptake (RAI)
> Triiodothyronine uptake (T_3)
> Protein-bound serum iodide (PBI)

Skin Tests

> Tuberculin test
> Schick test (for diphtheria)
> Coccidioidin test
> > (for coccidioidomycosis)
> Histoplasmin test (for histoplasmosis)

Agglutination Tests

> Blood typing
> Pregnancy determinations (on urine)

Syphilis Tests

> Flocculation (VDRL)
> Rapid Plasmin Reagin (RPR)
> Reiter protein complement fixation
> > (RPCF)

Urine Tests

> Corticosteroids determination
> Creatinine
> 17 Ketosteroid excretion
> PSP excretion
> Glucose (glucose tolerance tests)

Blood Hormones

> Adrenocorticotropin
> Androgens

Corticosteroids
Thyrotropin

Coagulation Tests

Bleeding time
Clotting time
Coagulation time
Prothrombin time

SUMMARY

There are many diagnostic procedures and tests that can not be done in the physician's office due to the elaborate equipment and the technical competence required to run the tests. For this reason, many diagnostic procedures are done outside the physicians office in a hospital, clinic, or laboratory.

The medical assistant should be familiar with the diagnostic tests that are frequently ordered by the physician. She must also be able to make the necessary arrangements for having those tests done, and must be sure that the patient is properly instructed about the test and preparation for it.

SUGGESTED ACTIVITIES

- Discuss why different physicians would be concerned with different types of diagnostic procedures.
- Make a list of available resources that provide detailed information about various diagnostic tests.
- Discuss several ways to increase knowledge of diagnostic procedures through everyday activities at school or work.

REVIEW

A. Complete the following statements.

1. A highly specialized area that is concerned with radioisotopes is _____.

2. An example of the function of pathology is the study of a _____ _____ or small tissue sample.

3. The study of secretions or body fluids takes place in a _____ _____.

B. Select the diagnostic tests from Column 2 which correspond with the proper classification in Column 1.

Column 1	Column 2
____ 1. RAI	a. Skin test
____ 2. PSP	b. Blood hormone
____ 3. Serum cholesterol	c. Renal function test
____ 4. Creatinine	d. GI tract test
____ 5. VDRL	e. Agglutination tests
____ 6. Androgens	f. Syphillis tests
____ 7. Bleeding time	g. Endocrine tests
____ 8. Blood typing	h. Pathology tests
____ 9. Schick test	i. Liver function tests
____ 10. Gastric pH	j. Coagulation tests
	k. Urine tests

Unit 35 Radiologic Examinations

OBJECTIVES

After completing this unit, the student should be able to

- Cite the dangers of exposure to X rays.
- Identify the precautions used to avoid overexposure to radiation from X rays.
- Prepare patients for radiologic examinations.

Radiologic examinations refer to the study of internal structures by the use of roentgen rays, or X rays. *X rays* are waves of energy that proceed outward from the source of the energy. They are electromagnetic and occupy a space in the electromagnetic spectrum. These waves are classified according to wavelength. All electromagnetic waves travel through space at about 186,000 miles per second. However, X rays have very short wavelengths. This short wavelength is the reason why X rays can go through materials that would reflect light rays.

DANGERS AND PRECAUTIONS

The ability to penetrate matter makes the use of X rays beneficial in medicine, both diagnostically and therapeutically. However, these radiologic examinations are potentially dangerous. When briefly directed at an area, X rays are capable of leaving an imprint of the structures that they passed through on a special film.

When X rays are taken repeatedly or a person is exposed to the radiation for a longer period of time, tissue destruction is the result. This is the reason why they are not taken indiscriminately or often. There is now more deliberate control over the taking of frequent chest X rays, and the radiologic examinations of pregnant women due to the danger of injury to the unborn child or the mother.

Patients should always be asked if they have had X rays taken within the past month; if they have, the physician must be informed before another one is taken. A patient who has had as many as 2500 milliamperes should not receive more radiation until a complete blood count has been done. X rays first destroy soft tissues. Then the red and white blood cells are affected. Bone, nerve, and finally brain tissues are affected last by the radiation.

If the medical assistant is helping with the actual procedure, she must also be very careful about personal overexposure. Most physicians will have a technician on the office staff if many X rays are taken in the office. However, there are still some doctors who teach their medical assistants to take X rays.

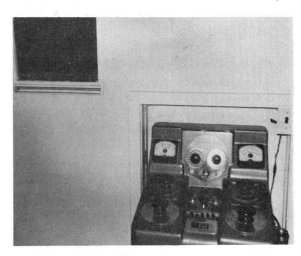

Fig. 35-1 **X-ray machine controls, and a window for viewing the patient.**

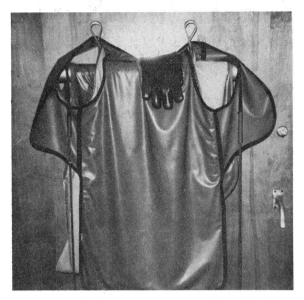

Fig. 35-2 A lead apron is worn as a safeguard against the penetration of X rays.

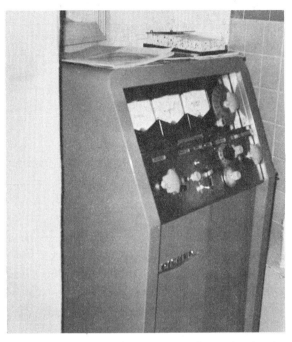

Fig. 35-3 X-ray controls must be located behind a lead wall or lead screen.

Any office that has x-ray equipment will also have a lead screen in the room which will prevent the rays from penetrating beyond the screen. X rays cannot pass through lead. The assistant must always stand behind this lead screen while an X ray is being taken. She should also wear a lead apron since X rays can scatter. The controls for operation of the machine will also be located behind the screen.

In addition, the assistant should wear a badge that will measure the amount of radiation to which she has been exposed. These badges must be processed once a week to determine if radiation has been absorbed. No more than about 3/10 roentgen may be absorbed weekly. A *roentgen* is the unit that is used for measuring x-ray dosage.

PATIENT PREPARATION

As in any other procedure, the patient must be told about the procedure to be done. Most people are familiar with the x-ray procedure and are not unduly anxious about it. However, there may be some people who have never had an X ray taken they will need reassurance. Do not forget that routine procedures that are very familiar to the medical assistant, can be extremely frightening to a person who is having them done for the first time. If specific questions about the dangers of radiation are asked, the patient should be referred to the physician.

The patient is escorted to the dressing room and instructed to remove clothing from the body area which is to be x-rayed. The patient must have privacy for undressing unless assistance is needed. Most physicians prefer having the patient completely undressed except for a gown which opens down the back.

All metals must be removed from the field to be x-rayed. Jewelry, hair pins, eyeglasses and any other such objects must be safely removed and put in a safe place until the procedure is completed. Necklaces, chains, and medals must be removed as metal imprints could lead to a false reading. The completed X ray has to be as clear as possible in order to help reach an accurate diagnosis.

Some patients will require assistance to get up on the x-ray table. A footstool should be available and used by all patients. Some patients will also need help in assuming the necessary positions. Always keep in mind that the patient may be in pain and the positions that must be assumed may cause the patient even more discomfort. Make the patient as comfortable as possible and remember that the x-ray table is often cold as well as very hard. Use a lightweight blanket to cover the patient, if necessary.

Equipment such as an emesis basin, ammonia ampules, and washcloths should be kept at hand; some patients may become nauseated or faint during the procedure due to anxiety or discomfort. Keep a very close watch on all patients for signs of physical or emotional distress.

X-RAY EXAMINATIONS

When taking films of bones, the patient must first be placed in the position that will give the best visibility of the affected part. In addition to the bones of the body, other types of tissues can be x-rayed. In some cases, tissues require special preparation. Although chest X rays do not require special preparation, they are taken at a setting of higher intensity and penetrating power than that used for x-ray examination of extremities.

Other types of soft tissues must be contrasted with a radiopaque material so that the tissues will be visible on the developed film. These radiopaque materials are called *contrast media* and may be administered to the patient in different ways. Some contrast media is given intravenously in the form of dyes. This preparation is *always* injected by the physician since some people have adverse reactions to the dyes; these reactions may range from mild discomfort to death if the proper action is not taken immediately. The assistant should never administer this type of contrast media.

Some preparations are taken internally through the digestive tract in order to film certain organs. *Barium sulfate* is frequently used to examine the gastrointestinal tract; it is a specially flavored preparation that the patient drinks. Still films may be made at given intervals to follow the progression of the barium or the physician may view the progress of the barium by *fluoroscopy*. This is a special technique for viewing the body's internal action and tissues while in motion. The *radiologist* is a physician who specializes in the field of diagnostic and therapeutic X rays.

Barium sulfate may also be administered as an enema to film the lower intestinal tract. Preparation for this X ray may take place in the office just before the X rays are taken.

The gallbladder, the kidneys, the uterus and fallopian tubes, and other tissues or organs may be x-rayed with special preparations. The assistant should keep a card file listing each procedure, the necessary preparation, and the purpose of the procedure until she is thoroughly familiar with the techniques and the patient preparation.

While some physicians will use standard equipment for making films of bones and/or chest X rays, the radiologic examinations which require contrast media will be done in the hospital or clinic. Professionally trained people are needed for these procedures.

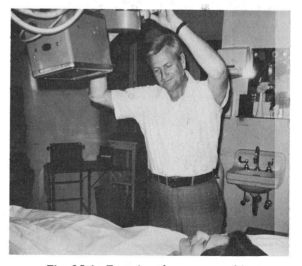

Fig. 35-4 Focusing the x-ray machine.

If the procedure is to be done in a setting other than the physician's office, the assistant must phone the clinic or hospital and make an appointment for the patient. At this time she checks the necessary preparation. The patient must be informed of the time, the place, and any advance preparation he must make before reporting to the clinic or hospital. It is the duty of the assistant to be sure that all necessary preparations are made. Keeping a card file is very helpful to be sure that preparations are not overlooked.

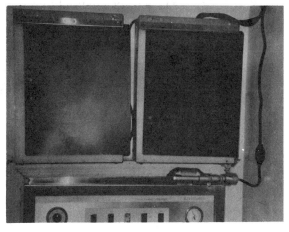
Fig. 35-5 Example of a viewing screen.

SUMMARY

Radiologic examinations (X rays) are potentially dangerous electromagnetic waves that penetrate tissue as well as most other materials with the exception of lead. Special precautions must be taken for the patient's protection as well as the working personnel.

The assistant must insure the patient's protection and comfort during radiologic procedures. She must also be certain that the patient is properly prepared for the procedure that is to be done.

The medical assistant's duties are limited to preparing the patient for x-ray procedures and assisting during the procedure, if necessary. If the patient is to have the films made in another facility, the assistant must schedule with that facility and be sure the patient has all the necessary instructions before the X rays are taken.

No assistant should take any X rays without special training and permission from the physician. She must never attempt to diagnose. Any questions from the patient should be referred to the physician. Diagnosing and determining what to tell the patient is the legal and professional duty of the physician only.

SUGGESTED ACTIVITIES

- Make arrangements to invite a radiologist to speak to the class on x-ray technique and its diagnostic and therapeutic uses.
- Invite an x-ray technician to discuss the special training required to become a radiologic technician.
- Visit an x-ray department or clinic and observe how they are made and developed.

REVIEW

Select the answer that best completes each statement.

1. X rays are both beneficial and potentially dangerous due to

   a. their ability to penetrate solid matter.
   b. their very short wavelength.
   c. their ability to penetrate matter rather than reflect off it as light rays do.
   d. all of these.
   e. none of these.

2. Lead screens are used in rooms with x-ray equipment to

   a. diffuse X rays.   d. absorb X rays.
   b. eliminate X rays.   e. none of these.
   c. stop X rays.

3. Badges are worn by persons working around X rays primarily to

   a. prevent X rays from penetrating the body.
   b. measure the amount of radiation that has been absorbed.
   c. determine how many milliamperes the assistant has received.
   d. identify the person as an employee of the x-ray department.
   e. all of the above.

4. If a patient has had X rays in the previous month, certain precautions must be taken. When should blood tests be taken before more X rays are made?

   a. if the patient has had 3/10 roentgens.
   b. if the patient has had 2500 milliamperes of radiation.
   c. if the patient has already had tissue destruction.
   d. all of the above.
   e. none of the above.

5. X rays may be taken of

   a. bones.   d. blood vessels.
   b. soft tissues.   e. all of these.
   c. organs.

6. Excessive exposure to X rays can result in

   a. superficial tissue destruction.
   b. internal tissue destruction.
   c. bone destruction and degeneration.
   d. destruction of red and white blood cells.
   e. all of the above.

7. Which of the following radiopaque materials may *not* be administered by the medical assistant?

   a. barium sulfate for a gastrointestinal series.
   b. dyes given intravenously.
   c. barium enemas.
   d. oral medications that are absorbed by specific organs of the body.
   e. all of the above.

8. The physician that specializes in radiology is called

   a. a radiologist.   d. all of these.
   b. a technologist.   e. none of these.
   c. a technician.

9. Overexposure to X rays can result in

    a. mental disorders.   d. tissue damage and degeneration.

    b. blood disorders.   e. both a and c.

    c. emotional disturbances.   f. both b and d.

10. Contrast media may be administered

    a. by mouth.   d. intramuscularly.

    b. rectally.   e. all except b.

    c. intravenously.   f. all except d.

11. The unit that is used for measuring x-ray dosage is

    a. milliliter.   c. cubic centimeter.

    b. amperes.   d. roentgen.

12. An excessive amount of x-ray radiation first destroys

    a. red and white blood cells.   c. soft tissues.

    b. bone tissue.   d. brain and nerve tissue.

Unit 36 Electrocardiography

OBJECTIVES

After completing this unit, the student should be able to

- Identify structures of the heart which are involved in following the course of an electrical impulse.
- Indicate placement of the six standard chest leads.
- Explain what takes place during depolarization and repolarization.
- Relate the lead circuits of EKG's to the correct electrode combinations.

The electrocardiogram is a reading obtained by a special apparatus called an electrocardiography machine (EKG machine). This machine is a direct writing instrument that measures the small electrical currents produced in the body during the cardiac cycle.

Electrical currents are produced by muscular contractions of the cardiac muscles. These currents are picked up by electrodes that are applied to various parts of the body and transmitted to the EKG machine. The machine relays the currents to a heated stylus that marks the signals onto a specially treated roll of EKG graph paper. A positive deflection of the stylus indicates that a current is moving toward the electrodes. A negative deflection indicates that the current is moving away from the electrodes. These deflections or waves are known as P, Q, R, S, and T waves. Their arrangement helps the physician determine the condition of the heart.

CARDIAC ACTIVITY

The medical assistant must thoroughly review the anatomy of the heart. In addition to the structural anatomy, the medical assistant

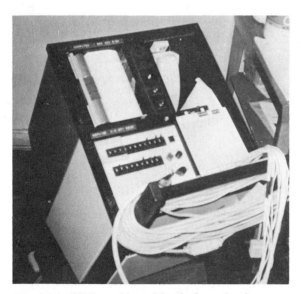

Fig. 36-1 EKG machine with telephone hookup to a computer center.

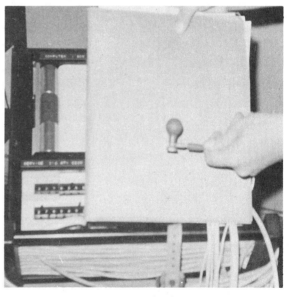

Fig. 36-2 Electrode for an EKG.

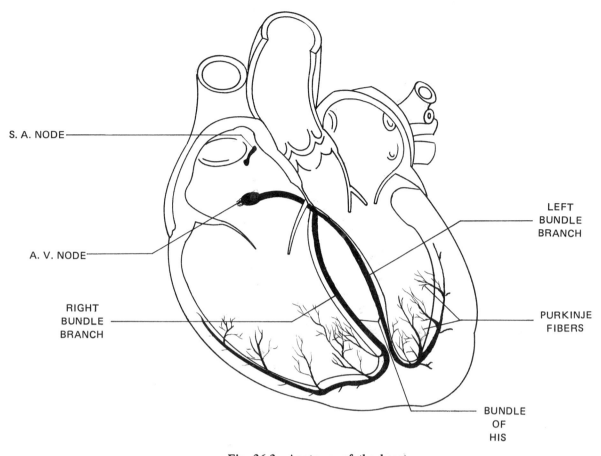

S. A. NODE

A. V. NODE

RIGHT
BUNDLE
BRANCH

LEFT
BUNDLE
BRANCH

PURKINJE
FIBERS

BUNDLE
OF
HIS

Fig. 36-3 Anatomy of the heart.

should be familiar with the electrical pathways and circuits of the cardiac cycle.

The contraction of the atria is excited by an impulse that is generated in the sinoatrial (S.A.) node which is sometimes referred to as the pacemaker of the cardiac cycle. As this electrical impulse *excites the atria,* a *P wave* is produced on the graph. The impulse then passes through the atrioventricular (A.V.) node and down the Bundle of His where it spreads through right and left bundle branches to the Purkinje fibers. These fibers excite the muscles of the ventricles and cause them to contract. This part of the cycle is called *depolarization* and is represented on the graph as the *QRS complex* or waves. The actual contraction of the ventricles occurs during the *repolarization* phase and is represented by the *ST waves.*

Occasionally, the *T* wave will be followed by a *U* wave which is not yet completely understood.

EKG LEADS

In order to measure a complete cardiac cycle's electrical circuit, electrodes are attached to the patient so that the electrical impulses may be monitored and recorded. The means of connecting the EKG machine to the patient's electrical circuit is by lead wires connected to the electrodes on the patient.

When the electrodes are attached to both the patient and the lead wires (connected to the EKG machine) the electrical currents pass from the left shoulder down the left arm, out the lead wire to and through the EKG machine, then through the lead wire to the

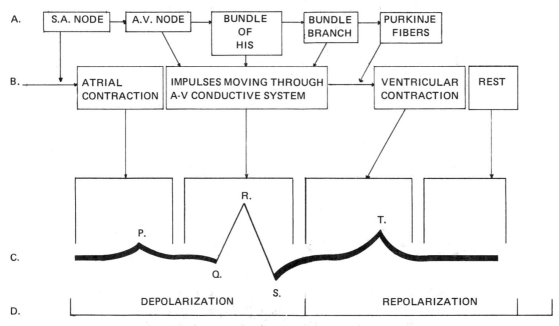

Fig. 36-4 Diagrammatic representation of cardiac impulses on EKG tracing. A. Course of electrical impulses. B. Cardiac muscle reaction to impulses. C. EKG tracing of impulse waves. D. Phases of cardiac cycle.

right arm, up the right shoulder and through the chest to the left shoulder. This makes up a complete circuit and the various parts of the cardiac electrical impulse cycle is recorded on the graph. This pathway is known as lead 1, figure 36-5.

The various combinations of the impulses transmitted by the electrodes have definite designations and these designations must be learned. The lead designations are

Lead 1	. .	right arm and left arm.	
Lead 2	. .	right arm and left leg.	*Limb*
Lead 3	. .	left arm and left leg.	*Leads*
Lead CR	. .	chest and right arm.	
Lead CL	. .	chest and left arm.	*Precordial*
Lead CF	. .	chest and left leg.	*Leads*
Lead AVR	.	right arm and central terminal (combined potentials of left leg and left arm).	
Lead AVL	.	left arm and central terminal (combined potentials of left leg and right arm).	*Unipolar Leads*
Lead AVF	.	left leg and central terminal (combined potentials of right and left arm).	
Lead V	. .	chest and central terminal (combined potential of the right arm, left arm, and left leg).	

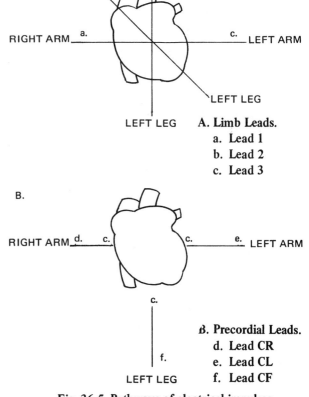

A. Limb Leads.
a. Lead 1
b. Lead 2
c. Lead 3

B.

B. Precordial Leads.
d. Lead CR
e. Lead CL
f. Lead CF

Fig. 36-5 Pathways of electrical impulses.

When a *unipolar* lead is identified, the exploring electrode is listed first and the indifferent electrode is listed last.

The chest or precordial leads must be very carefully placed by *exact* application of the chest electrode at the following positions, figure 36-6.

Lead V$_1$ . . . . fourth intercostal space immediately to the right of the sternum.

Lead V$_2$ . . . . fourth intercostal space immediately to the left of the sternum.

Lead V$_3$ . . . . midway between the electrode in Lead V$_2$ and Lead V$_4$.

Lead V$_4$ . . . . left fifth intercostal space at the midclavicular line.

Lead V$_5$ . . . . left anterior axillary line on the same level as Lead V$_4$.

Lead V$_6$ . . . . left midaxillary line at the level of V$_4$.

The doctor will determine what chest leads he wishes to use; all leads are marked on the tracing by depressing the Lead Marker button on the EKG machine. Doctors will use different codes according to their own preference. However, one code frequently used and recommended is shown on page 212.

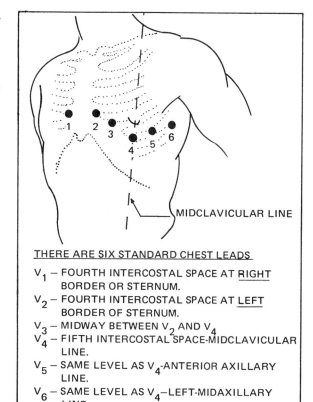

MIDCLAVICULAR LINE

THERE ARE SIX STANDARD CHEST LEADS

V$_1$ – FOURTH INTERCOSTAL SPACE AT <u>RIGHT</u> BORDER OR STERNUM.
V$_2$ – FOURTH INTERCOSTAL SPACE AT <u>LEFT</u> BORDER OF STERNUM.
V$_3$ – MIDWAY BETWEEN V$_2$ AND V$_4$
V$_4$ – FIFTH INTERCOSTAL SPACE-MIDCLAVICULAR LINE.
V$_5$ – SAME LEVEL AS V$_4$-ANTERIOR AXILLARY LINE.
V$_6$ – SAME LEVEL AS V$_4$–LEFT-MIDAXILLARY LINE.

Fig. 36-6 Conventional precordial lead positions.

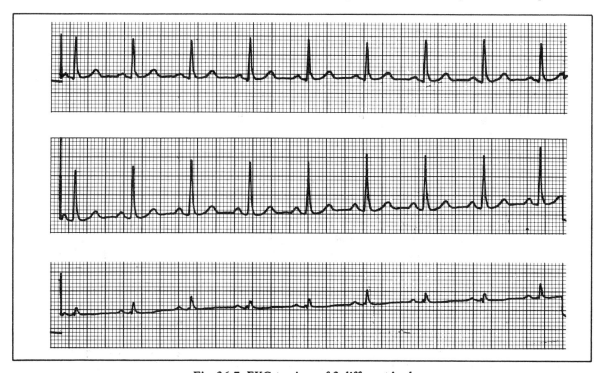

Fig. 36-7 EKG tracings of 3 different leads.

Lead 1	1 dot	.
Lead 2	2 dots	. .
Lead 3	3 dots	. . .
Lead CR	1 dot 1 dash 1 dot	. - .
Lead CL	1 dot 1 dash 2 dots	. - . .
Lead CF	1 dot 1 dash 3 dots	. - . . .
Lead AVR	1 dash	-
Lead AVL	2 dashes	- -
Lead AVF	3 dashes	- - -
Lead V_1	1 dash and 1 dot	- .
Lead V_2	1 dash and 2 dots	- . .
Lead V_3	1 dash and 3 dots	- . . .
Lead V_4	1 dash and 4 dots	- . . . .
Lead V_5	1 dash and 5 dots	- . . . . .
Lead V_6	1 dash and 6 dots	- . . . . . .

PREPARATION OF THE EKG MACHINE

Before running an EKG tracing on the patient, the machine must be checked for *standardization*. The machine must be properly *grounded* and the temperature of the stylus adjusted, if necessary, to provide a *dark baseline* on the tracing paper.

The machine must be allowed to warm up for at least 2 minutes if it is an older model. The newer models are ready to run in only a few seconds. Check to be sure the patient cable is connected to the machine as well as the lead wires.

Press the standardization button on the machine. One centimeter is equal to 10 millimeter lines on the tracing paper. *If the deflection of the stylus needle on the graph paper is more or less than one centimeter, the machine must be adjusted.* One centimeter of deflection for each millivolt of heart potential is accepted as the standard. This enables physicians anywhere to compare tracings from any EKG machine.

After checking the standardization, check to be sure the machine is properly grounded and then make sure a good baseline appears on the tracing paper. If the line is not clear or too heavy, adjust the temperature of the stylus accordingly so that a distinct black line is achieved. Be sure the stylus is centered in the middle of the tracing paper before beginning the patient tracing.

All EKG machines are very similar but the instruction manual should be studied and the assistant should make several practice tracings before running an EKG on a patient. This is an extremely important diagnostic test and should be accurately performed in every detail.

TAKING AN EKG

The patient must be relaxed and lying quietly in a warm, quiet room without distractions. The sheet covering the patient is turned back to expose the arms and legs for the placing of the electrodes.

A small amount of electrode jelly (enough to cover the surface of the skin where the electrode is to be) is rubbed onto the area using a 2" x 2" gauze square. The electrode surface is also covered with the electrode jelly and placed directly over the lubricated area of the skin. The electrode straps are fastened around the extremity to secure the electrodes and hold them firmly in place. Be careful not to spread the jelly from one area to another. To prevent this, use separate gauze square for each electrode application. Do not pull the electrode straps to tight, just tight enough to hold the electrode in place. Both the electrodes and the lead wires are marked or coded to ensure that they are placed on the correct extremity. For correct placement, the medical assistant should follow these steps:

- The right arm electrode is placed on the inner area of the right forearm.

- The left arm electrode is placed on the inner area of the left forearm.

- The right leg electrode is placed on the inner area of the right leg near the calf.

- The left leg electrode is placed on the inner area of the left leg near the calf.

- Be sure that all electrodes are making good contact.

• Until the assistant becomes proficient at applying the electrodes, she should use about 1/2 inch of electrode jelly for each application to ensure good surface contact.

• Placement of the chest electrode will vary according to which lead is desired but the technique for placement is the same as for the limb leads.

• After placement of the electrodes, check again to be certain that the proper lead wires have been connected to the electrodes.

The assistant should be thoroughly familiar with the EKG machine that she is using before attempting to take an EKG. All machines have instructions that explain the maintenance and operation of that particular machine.

SUMMARY

The medical assistant must be thoroughly familiar with the equipment that she is working with. In order to run a good EKG tracing on a patient, the assistant must be sure the patient is comfortable and relaxed. The electrodes must be properly in place with good contact. The electrodes must also be connected to the correct lead wires and the lead wires connected to the EKG machine. The patient cable must also be connected. The EKG machine must be checked for standardization.

The assistant must know the proper position for the electrodes as well as the leads resulting from the various combinations of the electrodes. She must also know the code that is used in the physician's office.

SUGGESTED ACTIVITIES

• Make arrangements to invite a cardiologist to speak on the importance of taking good electrocardiograms.

• Inspect some completed, well-coded EKG tracings. Identify the P wave, the QRS complex, the S and T waves.

• Make a drawing of the heart and correlate the EKG waves with the parts of the heart.

• Observe the proper way to apply the electrodes to the patient. Practice applying electrodes.

• After reading the instruction manual for the EKG machine, practice preparing the patient for an EKG. With supervision, run a tracing on a classmate.

REVIEW

A. In the space provided by each description of a lead, place the correct name or number for that lead.

1. _____ left arm and left leg.
2. _____ chest and left leg.
3. _____ right arm and central terminal (combined potentials of the left leg and left arm).
4. _____ right arm and left leg.
5. _____ chest and left arm.

6. _____ right arm and left arm.

7. _____ left leg and central terminal consisting of combined potentials of the right and left arm.

8. _____ chest and central terminal (combined potentials of the right and left arm and the left leg).

9. _____ chest and right arm.

10. _____ left arm and central terminal (combined potentials of the left leg and right arm).

B. Fill in the correct chest lead number.

1. _____ the electrode is placed in the fourth intercostal space just to the left of the sternum.

2. _____ the electrode is placed between V_2 and V_4.

3. _____ the electrode is placed on the left anterior axillary line at the level of lead V_4.

4. _____ the electrode is placed on the left fifth intercostal space at the midclavicular line.

5. _____ the electrode is placed on the level of V_4 but on the left midaxillary line.

C. Study each code in the first column and select the appropriate lead from the list. Enter the answer in the blank which precedes each code.

Leads

1. _____ - -   Lead V_5
2. _____ .   Lead 1
3. _____ - . . . . . Lead CF
4. _____ . - .   Lead AVL
5. _____ . - . . .   Lead V_1
6. _____ . .   Lead AVF
7. _____ - .   Lead 3
8. _____ - - -   Lead CR
9. _____ -   Lead AVR
10. _____ . . .   Lead 2

D. Select the answer which best completes the statement.

1. The sinoatrial (S.A.) node generates an electrical impulse that stimulates the

a. ventricles.   c. Bundle of His.
b. atria.   d. Purkinje fibers.

2. The muscles of the ventricles are excited by the electrical impulses from the

a. ventricles.   c. Bundle of His.
b. atria.   d. Purkinje fibers.

3. The depolarization phase of the cardiac cycle is represented on the tracing by the

   a. P waves.   c. ST waves.
   b. QRS waves.   d. U waves.

4. Repolarization is represented on the tracing by the

   a. P waves.   c. ST waves.
   b. QRS waves.   d. U waves.

5. The pacemaker of the heart is the

   a. sinoatrial node.   c. Bundle of His.
   b. atrioventricular node. d. U wave.

6. Standardization of the EKG machine is done to check

   a. if the machine has warmed up for two minutes.
   b. if the stylus is deflected 10 millimeters when the button is pressed.
   c. if the stylus is centered in the middle of the graph paper.
   d. if a good baseline is present.

7. Lead V is a
   a. limb lead.   c. bipolar lead.
   b. precordial lead.   d. unipolar lead.

Self-Evaluation Test 6

Select the answers that best complete the following statements.

1. The reading that is obtained by a special apparatus which measures and records the electrical currents produced in the body is called an

   a. electrocardiography. c. electroencephalogram.
   b. electrocardiogram.   d. none of these.

2. A positive deflection of the EKG stylus indicates a

   a. QRS wave.
   b. current moving toward the electrode.
   c. ST complex.
   d. current moving away from the electrode.

3. The electrical impulse that arises in the sinoatrial node results in

   a. the contraction of the ventricles.
   b. the relaxation of the atria.
   c. the stimulation and contraction of the atria.
   d. the stimulation of the Bundle of His.

4. The passage of the electrical current through the A.V. node, down the Bundle of His, down the bundle branches, and to the Purkinje fibers is correlated on the EKG by

   a. the P wave.   c. the ST waves.
   b. the QRS complex. d. the U wave.

5. Lead 1, Lead 2, and Lead 3 are known or designated as the

   a. precordial leads. c. limb leads.
   b. unipolar leads.   d. indifferent leads.

6. Standardization of the EKG machine is done before each EKG is run to

   a. be sure the temperature of the stylus provides a good baseline.
   b. check to ensure adequate grounding of the machine.
   c. enable physicians anywhere to compare EKG tracings.
   d. none of the above.

7. The short wavelength of X rays makes them beneficial to medicine. This short wavelength also makes them

   a. potentially dangerous.
   b. difficult to contain.
   c. capable of penetrating most matter except lead.
   d. all of the above.

8. Since X rays destroy tissues and blood cells, a patient should have a complete blood count taken if he has recently received more than
   a. 25,000 milliamperes.   c. 2500 milliamperes.
   b. 3/10 ampere.   d. none of these.

9. Since X rays can and do scatter, the medical assistant must stand behind a lead screen when taking them. Another necessary, protective step is
   a. take no more than four X rays a day.
   b. use a·lead apron when working around X rays.
   c. have a complete blood count done weekly.
   d. all of the above.

10. The unit of measurement that is used to measure radiation dosage is the
    a. roentgen.   c. ampere.
    b. radiology.   d. milliampere.

11. Radiopaque material or contrast media is administered to the patient in order to make films of soft tissue. Which of the following methods is NOT used for the administration of contrast media?
    a. intramuscularly.   c. orally.
    b. intravenously.   d. rectally.

12. When the physician views the actions of internal organs and structures rather than still films, the process is known as
    a. radiography.   c. fluoroscopy.
    b. radiology.   d. all of these.

13. Excessive X rays first cause damage to
    a. the blood.   c. the mind.
    b. the soft tissues.   d. the bones.

14. If specialized laboratory studies were required to analyze tissue fluids, they would be done in the
    a. nuclear laboratory.   c. pathology department.
    b. clinical laboratory.   d. x-ray department.

15. The specialty area of laboratory studies involved with ionizing radiation and radioisotopes is called
    a. pathology.   c. nuclear medicine.
    b. radiology.   d. none of these.

16. An aid that is helpful to the medical assistant in preparing patients for diagnostic studies is
    a. memorize all of the tests that might be done.
    b. ask the doctor to give you the information that you need each time a test is scheduled.
    c. call the facility where the testing is to take place to get the information needed.
    d. keep an up-to-date card file.

17. The tuberculin test belongs in the category of

    a. skin testing.
    b. blood hormones.
    c. syphilis testing.
    d. none of these.

18. A gastrointestinal series is a diagnostic procedure that belongs in the general category of

    a. clinical laboratory studies.
    b. pathological studies.
    c. radiology studies.
    d. nuclear testing.

19. Which of the following tests would be placed in the category of endocrine system tests?

    a. radioactive iodine uptake.
    b. thymol turbidity.
    c. creatinine.
    d. PSP determination.

20. The arrangements for patient testing to be done outside the doctor's office are usually made by

    a. the physician.
    b. the medical assistant.
    c. the receptionist.
    d. the patient.

Section 7
Emergencies

Unit 37 Physical Crises

OBJECTIVES

After completing this unit, the student should be able to

- Identify what is meant by a crisis.

- Describe proper action to be taken in specific crises.

There will be occasions of physical crises in the doctor's office. A *crisis* is a time when immediate action must be taken; it is a decisive moment. Every adult should know proper emergency action; the assistant is no exception.

In group office practice, there will be a physician within reach in most instances; if one doctor is out, usually there are other physicians in the building. However, if a doctor is not immediately available and the emergency calls for immediate medical treatment, the assistant must make arrangements to get the patient to the hospital as soon as possible. This is a decision that the assistant must make and her judgment must be sound. Also, the medical assistant should know where her doctor may be located for emergencies. He will be able to meet the patient at the emergency room. The assistant must be prepared to deal with these situations in a competent, responsible manner; a patient's life may depend on it.

SHOCK

Shock occurs when the blood circulation has been disturbed to the extent where body functions are upset. It happens when the blood pressure is not adequate enough to force blood through the vital organs.

Shock can result from may causes. It may accompany physical injury, emotional crises, or other stress.

A patient who is in shock must be kept warm and the vital signs must be watched closely. He should be placed on a bed or treatment table with the feet elevated to encourage blood flow to the head.

Blankets are placed over the patient. *The pulse, respiration, and blood pressure are watched constantly and the physician kept informed.*

Never give an unconscious patient any liquids by mouth as the patient might aspirate the fluid into the lungs. If the patient is conscious and alert, a hot liquid such as coffee or tea may be given.

If these measures do not revive the patient, the physician may order a stimulant. He will administer the stimulant. If the doctor is not available and there is not another physician nearby, call an ambulance and send the patient to the nearest emergency center.

HEMORRHAGE

Hemorrhage refers to excessive loss of blood. Hemorrhage can result from a number of different causes. The first thing to do is to try to stop the bleeding regardless of the cause.

A hemorrhage from a wound can often be stopped by applying pressure bandages to the wound. If the hemorrhage is the result of damage to a large artery or vein, the area of the injury should be elevated and a pressure bandage applied. Many doctors today discourage the use of tourniquets except in the case of an amputation. Every effort should be made to stop the bleeding without the use of a tourniquet. If the bleeding is from an open wound, sterile technique must be maintained.

Nosebleed (epistaxis) may be stopped if pressure is applied to the anterior part of the nose while the patient is seated, with the head held forward. Ice applied to the bridge of the nose combined with pressure will usually stop or decrease the flow of blood until further measures may be taken by the doctor.

Uterine bleeding, if severe, is a very dangerous situation. The patient should be placed flat on a bed or treatment table, with the legs elevated slightly. The head should be lower than the legs if at all possible. The assistant should not attempt to pack the vagina with anything to stop the flow if there is medical help within the immediate area. Legal complications may arise if there is any suspicion of abortion or any injuries present due to an illegal abortion. The assistant could be blamed for injuries if she applied any type of packing for uterine bleeding. If lying down with the feet elevated does not decrease or stop the flow of blood, hospitalization will be required if a physician is not available.

FAINTING

Fainting is a temporary loss of consciousness. It is a fairly frequent occurrence and is easily dealt with in most cases.

The patient should be lying down. Loosen any tight clothing. Apply a cold cloth to the forehead. If necessary break an ammonia ampule, using gauze squares to do so, or saturate a gauze sponge with aromatics of ammonia and hold it briefly underneath the patient's nose. After regaining consciousness, the patient should be allowed to rest until he can stand upright without help. The patient's color should return and the pallor have gone before allowing a patient to leave.

If a patient feels faint but is not unconscious, have him bend forward from a sitting position with his head lowered between his knees. This will increase the blood flow to the head and often prevent fainting.

SEIZURES AND CONVULSIONS

A *seizure* is a spasm; a temporary disturbance in muscular coordination and control. Every office should have well-padded tongue blades in each room in case of seizures or convulsions. Two tongue blades are placed together and then wrapped with gauze and adhesive tape.

The padded tongue blade is put between a patient's teeth at the beginning of the convulsion in order to help keep the airway open and to prevent damage to the teeth and tissues of the mouth. *Do not attempt to restrain a patient during convulsions* as severe injuries or even fractures may result. Do not force the padded tongue blades into the patient's mouth if the jaws are set and the convulsion is in progress. Protect the patient as much as possible by pushing away any furniture and objects that might cause injury. Stay with the patient, holding the padded tongue blades between the teeth (crosswise) until the seizure passes. Someone should be sent for the doctor immediately. If a padded tongue blade is not handy, a handkerchief folded several times may be placed between the teeth, with the ends of the handkerchief protruding from both sides of the mouth. (A wallet may also be used in an emergency).

As soon as the seizure passes, the patient should be covered with a blanket and kept quiet until medical help arrives.

POISONING

A poison chart should be easily accessible in every office. Poison control centers are located in all larger cities. The telephone number of the poison control center should be posted in a prominent place near a phone in the office. While most poison ingestion cases will go directly to the hospital rather than the office, the number of the poison control center should be near to give to anyone needing it. Time is vital in poison ingestion. If the assistant receives a call about poison ingestion, she should ask what was taken and tell the caller to go straight to the hospital. If the caller does not know what poison was taken, emphasize that any opened bottles or cans near the patient should be taken with them. Call the hospital and tell them that a poison ingestion case is on the way. Inform the emergency room what substance was ingested if it is known.

If the physician is not in and cannot talk with the caller, and if the caller is more than a few minutes away from medical help, the medical assistant must try to find out what has been swallowed because immediate dilution or neutralization of the substance may save the life. If the substance is unknown, fluids such as milk or water should be forced on the patient as soon as possible. An attempt should be made to force vomiting by placing the fingers down the throat after the substance has been diluted. This should be done several times. CAUTION: Vomiting should not be forced if the poison is of a caustic nature as more tissue damage will occur.

Alkalies such as a dilution of baking soda in water should be given if the ingested poison is an acid. Milk and/or egg whites are antidotes for mineral poisoning such as nitrate of silver. If there is doubt about the type of substance ingested, rely on milk or water and force as much as possible down the patient if he is conscious. Get to a medical facility as soon as possible.

FRACTURES

If a fracture should occur in the office and the physician is not available, keep the patient still and lying down with blankets to prevent shock. The injured area should not be moved until competent help arrives. Call for an ambulance and stay with the patient until the ambulance arrives. Be sure that the injured area is properly supported during the transfer to the ambulance.

BURNS

Ice should be applied immediately to burns caused by heat. If ice is not available, cold water on the burn will help. Totally submerge the affected part in cold water if possible. If not, allow cold running water to flow over the area until ice can be obtained.

Chemical burns should have the chemical removed from the skin surface immediately by gently and quickly wiping off any excess and then rinsing in cold, clear water. If the burn was caused by an acid (except carbolic acid) apply a weak alkali like bicarbonate of soda. If the acid is carbolic acid, apply alcohol. Vinegar is applied to strong alkaline burns such as might result from potash, quicklime, or caustic soda.

CARDIAC ARREST

Should a patient suddenly stop breathing and you cannot find a pulse or heartbeat, get help immediately. Resuscitation must begin within minutes of the arrest to avoid permanent damage. Many medical assistants who are being trained in cardiopulmonary resuscitation are also receiving training in other emergency situations.

Do not try to administer emergency treatment unless you have been trained to do so. While help is on the way check to see that the patient's airway is not obstructed; if it is obstructed, try to remove the object, being careful not to push it further down the airway.

Position the patient flat on a hard surface and with the head turned slightly to one side. Loosen any tight or restrictive clothing. Cover the patient with a blanket. While waiting for medical help have someone look for a trained individual who is capable of giving cardiopulmonary resuscitation. Obviously, since saving a life may depend on knowledge of emergency action and immediate action, every medical assistant should learn how to give cardiopulmonary resuscitation. Courses are available in all communities. The local Red Cross chapter is one source of information about such courses.

SUMMARY

The medical assistant should be prepared to deal with many varied emergency situations in the absence of the doctor. She should be familiar with her doctor's methods of handling emergencies and keep this in mind at all time.

Should an emergency occur in the absence of the doctor, the assistant is responsible for the patient until she can get the patient to another medical facility or physician. Since many doctors' offices are grouped together or located nearby, there should be available help if needed.

Most emergencies will go directly to the emergency room of the nearest hospital rather than to the doctor's office. However, should emergencies present themselves, the assistant must be able to deal with them competently and professionally.

SUGGESTED ACTIVITIES

- Through role-playing, present various types of emergencies. Discuss the actions taken.

- Make arrangements to invite an emergency room physician to speak about emergencies that can be handled in the office and those that should go directly to the hospital.

- Contact the nearest poison control center. Make arrangements for a speaker to talk to the class. Request literature and other materials for class discussion.

REVIEW

A. Complete the following.

    1. Give an antidote for the following.

        a. nitrate of silver _____

        b. acid solutions _____

        c. unknown solution _____

    2. The three things that should be done for a patient having a seizure are:

        a. _____

        b. _____

        c. _____

3. The first thing that must be done in a case of hemorrhage is

_____

B. Briefly answer the questions.

1. In chemical burns, what is the first step of treatment?

2. What would be applied to a chemical burn caused by an alkali?

3. What would be applied to a chemical burn caused by carbolic acid?

4. If a chemical burn was caused by a strong acid other than carbolic acid, what would be applied?

5. In uterine bleeding, the assistant should not pack the vagina to stop the bleeding. Why?

6. If a patient does not respond to the treatment for shock that the assistant gives, what should be done?

Unit 38 Psychological Crises

OBJECTIVES

After completing this unit, the student should be able to

- Describe how to approach a hysterical patient.
- Given an example of a case of attempted suicide, state how to handle the situation.
- Develop an awareness of principles which underlie the care of patients with emotional problems.

Occasionally a medical assistant must deal with situations concerning psychological crises of patients. She must be able to function efficiently, calmly, and maturely in these situations, keeping the patient's well-being in mind at all times.

THE HYSTERICAL PATIENT

Hysteria can occur as the result of many things or a combination of occurrences and pressures. Hysteria is marked by an obvious loss of self-control; the problem-solving attitude and the manner of handling difficult situations are affected. These situations may present themselves to the patient in the home environment or may arise from anxiety and fear in the doctor's office. Regardless of the cause, a firm, understanding approach to a hysterical patient is necessary.

Hysteria may manifest itself in many different ways. Seldom will any two people react in the same way to difficult circumstances. The medical assistant must approach hysterical people with understanding and calmness. Often a sympathetic person will only cause a hysterical person to become more agitated. If the emotionally upset person can feel that someone is concerned, even though there is not approval of the emotional reaction, calmness may result so that the problem may

be discussed in a reasonable way. However, there will be times when more is needed than just calm understanding to quiet an agitated patient. The physician must handle this as he is far more experienced in dealing with severe emotional crises. Never, under any circumstances, should the patient be slapped to stop a hysterical outburst. Striking a patient could result in a lawsuit against both the doctor and the assistant. If the doctor cannot calm the patient, a sedative may be administered to quiet the patient so that communication may take place. Dealing with these types of situa-

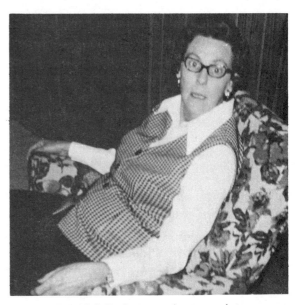

Fig. 38-1 Patient reacting to anxiety.

tions requires patience and understanding which come with maturity and experience.

ATTEMPTED SUICIDE

Should the medical assistant be faced with a case of attempted suicide, she should remember at all times that these cases can result in legal inquires. She should remain calm and composed and never be critical or condescending. This is a time of severe emotional turmoil for the family as well as the patient. A professional attitude should serve the assistant well in this situation as long as there is no appearance of indifference or aloofness. The physician will take appropriate action and do what is required for the patient. The assistant may be needed to assist the physician or to stay with the family. Do not say meaningless phrases or words to the family. Rather than sitting and sympathizing with the family, it is often more helpful to inquire if any phone calls could be made for them. Since all of the circumstances surrounding an attempted suicide are not known, do not make any moral judgments. If the patient is conscious, do not make any religious overtures to the family or the patient. Respect their wishes and do not force religious comfort on them as this could be extremely offensive to some people. Do not express any shock or dismay at circumstances involving attempted or successful suicides. The assistant must not pass judgment on patients in any circumstances.

THE EMOTIONALLY ILL PATIENT

Occasionally, the medical assistant will be working with emotionally disturbed or handicapped patients. Always remember that

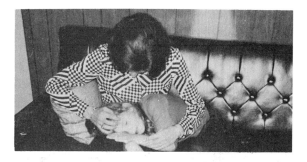

Fig. 38-2   A mother comforting a disturbed child.

they are ill and are not acting the way they do from choice. The medical assistant must be exceptionally patient and understanding. This is much easier to do if she remembers to put herself in the patient's or the family's place. Never show distaste or repulsion toward emotionally handicapped people. They can no more help themselves than can a physically ill person. They should be treated with the same respect and dignity as any other person. Compassion is a very necessary attribute of a medical assistant.

SUMMARY

In all cases of emotional crisis, the medical assistant must be understanding, calm, and compassionate. Each patient and each circumstance must be dealt with differently and intelligently. Never, under any circumstances, is the assistant to show or express distaste, disapproval, or condescension toward patients or families with an emotional crisis. The assistant may help both the family and the patient but she must know when the situation should be turned over to the physician. Common sense will often see the medical assistant through difficult situations involving emotional crises.

SUGGESTED ACTIVITIES

- With a classmate, role play the part of a medical assistant and a patient undergoing a psychological crisis. Follow the presentation with a class discussion.

- Make arrangements to have a psychiatrist or a psychologist speak to the class about emotional crises and how to deal with them.

- Make arrangements to have a seminar on attempted suicide and death. A minister, a clergyman, a policeman, and a psychologist or psychiatrist could be asked to participate as guest speakers.

REVIEW

Select the answer that best completes the following statements.

1. A distraught mother has brought her daughter into the office in her arms. The girl is about 14 years old and very groggy. The mother tells you that the girl has taken an overdose of tranquilizers and tried to take her own life. Which of the following actions would the medical assistant *NOT* take?

   a. Tell the physician immediately.
   b. Ask the mother if there is anyone that you can call for her, such as her husband or a friend.
   c. Ask the mother what occurred to cause such a terrible thing to happen.
   d. Prepare the treatment room for the patient.

2. A patient has just been told by the physician that she has cancer. The patient walks out of the doctor's office and starts crying and shaking in the reception room. Which of the following would the assistant do first?

   a. Loudly call out for the doctor.
   b. Have the patient sit down in the reception room while you go to tell the doctor.
   c. Lead the patient to one of the treatment rooms and send someone else for the doctor while you stay with the patient.
   d. Take the patient to a place where she can lie down and then go tell the doctor what has happened.

3. An emotionally disturbed child is becoming very agitated in the reception room while waiting to be seen by the doctor. Select the best course of action for the assistant to take.

   a. Ask the mother to take the child outside for awhile.
   b. Ask the mother if she would like to take the child to an empty room and see if she can quiet him down.
   c. Immediately take the child to the physician.
   d. Inform the doctor of the child's increasing agitation and ask the mother if there is anything that you can do to help.

Self-Evaluation Test 7

Select the answers that best complete the following statements.

1. If a patient or person is becoming hysterical, sympathy often will cause the hysterical person to

   a. calm down.
   b. burst into tears and become more agitated.
   c. become more rational and easier to deal with.
   d. none of the above.

2. Hysteria will not manifest itself in the same manner in all people because

   a. everyone is basically alike.
   b. most people will respond to similar situations in a similar manner.
   c. people react to situations in different ways.
   d. people are unpredictable in every way.

3. If a calm, competent, understanding medical assistant cannot quiet an upset patient who is bordering on hysteria, she should

   a. be very firm with the patient and tell him that he must calm down or leave the office immediately.
   b. ask the physician to handle the situation.
   c. appeal to the patient to please quiet down so as not to disturb the other patients in the office.
   d. sympathetically, take the patient to a secluded room or area.

4. When an attempted suicide occurs in a family, the family is usually

   a. embarrassed about the incident.
   b. concerned about the outcome of the attempt.
   c. worried about any legal implications.
   d. all of the above.

5. In the event of an attempted suicide, the assistant can

   a. call her own minister.
   b. ask the family who their minister is so that she can call him.
   c. offer to make any phone calls.
   d. ask if there is anyone the family would like to have with them and offer to call them.

6. Keeping the patient warm, dry, and with the head lower than the feet while monitoring the vital signs is standard treatment for

   a. fractures.   c. cardiac arrest.
   b. shock.   d. convulsions.

7. If profuse bleeding occurs, the first step taken to stop it would be to

   a. apply a tourniquet.
   b. apply a pressure bandage.
   c. elevate the hemorrhaging part.
   d. apply a tight packing to the wound.

8. The medical term for nosebleed is

   a. localized hemorrhage.   c. aspiration.
   b. epistaxis.   d. internal hemorrhage.

9. A padded tongue blade should be kept within easy reach in all doctor's offices in case of

   a. epistaxis.   c. shock.
   b. hemorrhage.   d. convulsions.

10. In the case of internal poisoning by an unknown agent, the patient should be made to

    a. vomit immediately.
    b. drink large amounts of a slightly alkaline solution.
    c. drink large amounts of a slightly acid solution.
    d. drink large amounts of water or milk.

11. The agency that should be immediately notified of a poison ingestion case is the

    a. doctor's office.   c. local poison control center.
    b. hospital emergency room.   d. police department.

12. If a patient sustains a fracture in the doctor's office and the doctor is out, the medical assistant should

    a. splint the fracture until it can be set by the doctor.
    b. take X rays so that time can be saved and the X rays will be ready for the doctor.
    c. call an ambulance and keep the patient still and warm until it arrives.
    d. leave the patient covered with a blanket while you find another doctor to see the patient.

13. In the case of burns caused by intense heat,

    a. apply the appropriate antidote.   c. rinse the area first.
    b. apply ice immediately.   d. none of these.

14. A chemical burn caused by carbolic acid should be rinsed with running water and then

    a. a solution of bicarbonate of soda is applied.
    b. a vinegar solution is applied.
    c. alcohol is applied.
    d. caustic soda is applied.

Appendix

Introduction to the Specialty Areas

The medical assistant will find that there are many different types of medical specialties and that each one involves different duties.

The practice of medicine is generally divided into two broad areas: *general medical practice* and *specialty areas*. General medical practice covers all areas of medicine and the physician who practices in this area is called a general practitioner (GP). The physicians who practice in a specialty area are known by the type of specialty that they practice; for example, an obstetrician specializes in obstetrics, a cardiologist specializes in the diseases of the heart.

The field of medicine has become so very large and comprehensive that it is almost impossible for one man or woman to learn everything there is to know. Therefore, the general practitioner must know about all areas of medicine in some detail while the specialist is an expert about his specialty and knows it in great detail. The practice of medicine is a group effort in many ways. The general practitioner can and does diagnose and treat disorders and diseases of all kinds but he also refers patients with special needs or problems to the specialist. After the problem has been solved or is in the process of solution, the specialist refers the patient back to the general practitioner for continued care.

A brief introduction to the specialties follows. General information is given in order to acquaint the student with each of the specialties.

CARDIOLOGY AND INTERNAL MEDICINE

Cardiology is the study and science of treating diseases and disorders of the heart. The physician who practices cardiology is known as a cardiologist.

The cardiologist studies the structure and function of the heart, determines the presence of abnormalities or disorders, what those disorders are, and what is the best method of treating those disorders to return the patient to an active and healthy life.

The cardiologist is both a diagnostician and a clinical therapist. For this reason, the equipment found in a cardiologist's office is directly related to necessary diagnostic procedures and treatment. Obviously, some of this equipment will differ from that found in other types of offices.

The medical assistant would also be expected to have different skills than those required in other types of offices. Some of the basic skills will be used but there will also be additional skills required in order to assist the cardiologist in his practice.

Internal medicine is the practice of diagnosing and treating disorders of the internal organs. The physician who practices internal medicine is called an internist. The title, *internist,* is not to be confused with *intern.* An *intern* is a graduate of medical school, who is serving a required period of clinical training before he can become a physician licensed to practice medicine.

The *internist* is a physician who has specialized in one area of medicine after completing all the requirements of being a medical doctor. He has additional training in his specialty beyond what is required to practice general medicine.

A medical assistant who works for an internist is required to do more EKGs, laboratory, and x-ray work than in other types of offices.

DERMATOLOGY AND ALLERGY

The study of diseases and disorders of the skin or integumentary system is called *dermatology*. The physician who practices dermatology is a dermatologist.

The causes of skin disorders range from allergies and emotional disturbances to congenital lesions and malignant tumors. The therapy is varied and takes on many forms.

Problems which arise from dermatologic disorders require special understanding and care because many disorders result in disfigurement and permanent damage. Therefore, a dermatologist is concerned not only with the physical problems but the emotional and psychological problems that can arise from these disorders.

The medical assistant who works for a dermatologist must be an understanding, compassionate individual who can relate to people easily. She must be the kind of person who does not allow unsightly skin disorders to make her uncomfortable. The dermatology patient needs support and understanding from the physician and his assistants as well as medical care for the skin disorder.

Allergy is referred to as a state of altered immunological reactivity that results in injury to the body as in the case of asthma, allergic rhinitis (hay fever) and gastrointestinal reactions. In more simple terms, it is an abnormal sensitivity to substances that are ordinarily harmless to the average person. The physician who practices the diagnosis and treatment of allergical conditions is an allergist.

EAR, NOSE, AND THROAT

When a physician specializes in the treatment of the ears, nose, and throat, he is involved in the specialty referred to as ENT (ear, nose, and throat).

Otology is the study of disorders of the ear. If the physician specializes exclusively in otology, he is an otologist.

Laryngology is the study of disorders and treatment of the larynx, pharynx, nasopharynx, and tracheobronchial tree.

There are many disorders that are diagnosed and treated by either a specialist in the field of ENT or an otologist or laryngologist. Sinusitis, epistaxis, tonsilitis, adenoiditis, and deviated septums are a few of the conditions that would be treated by a specialist in this field. The conditions treated might be caused by allergic reactions, congenital malformations, infectious disorders, or trauma.

ENDOCRINOLOGY

The study of the endocrine system and its disorders is known as *endocrinology* and is practiced by an endocrinologist. There are many classifications of endocrine disorders. The consequences of the disorders of the ductless glands are usually due either to overproduction or an underproduction of hormones. This imbalance of hormonal production can cause widespread pathological conditions throughout the body as well as mental and emotional disorders.

Endocrinology is concerned with ductless glands such as the thyroid gland, the parathyroid glands, the adrenal gland, and the pituitary gland. The hormones produced by these glands regulate many body functions as well as normal growth and reproduction. Most of the diagnostic studies are done in the clinical laboratory. Some metabolic testing may be done in the office.

GERONTOLOGY

Gerontology is the study of aging and its effects. Disorders that accompany the aging process are also studied. Care of the aged is known as *geriatrics*. Actually, this is a specialty area that includes other specialties since the process of aging affects all of the organs of the body and both physical and mental processes.

At one time, the life expectancy was as short as 30 or 35 years. Now, one may expect to live well beyond 70 to 80 years of age and still experience an active, rewarding life. This greatly increased life expectancy has opened up the specialty of gerontology and the care of the older patient.

The older person has many problems directly related to aging which are different from the disorders and diseases treated by other areas of medicine. Some of these problems are not truly disorders or diseases but are simply the results of growing older. Therefore, a large part of the practice of gerontology or geriatrics is preventive and maintenance medicine.

NEUROLOGY

The study of *neurology* is the study of disorders of cognitive, sensory, or psychomotor functions. The physician practicing neurology is a neurologist.

This is a complicated specialty and a very important one since even the simplest activities demand coordination within the nervous system. A simple act like feeding oneself requires extremely complicated coordination within the neurological system as well as with the muscular, structural, and cerebral functions of the body.

Patients need reassurance and instruction about the neurological exam. This type of examination is quite different than the routine physical exam. The physician uses percussion hammers, sharp and blunt instruments, tuning forks and various tests to determine the patient's balance and mental orientation.

Some common neurological disorders are meningitis, Parkinson's disease, epilepsy, multiple sclerosis, myasthenia gravis, and encephalitis. Neurological disorders can also result from trauma, congenital disorders, infectious processes and causes of unknown origins.

OBSTETRICS AND GYNECOLOGY

Obstetrics is the practice of medicine that is involved with pregnancy, labor, delivery, and postpartum care. The specialist is an obstetrician.

The obstetrician checks the pregnant woman often in order to assure the maintenance of good health, and to find and treat any problems that might arise during the pregnancy.

When the woman goes into labor, the obstetrician carefully follows the progress of labor and delivers the newborn baby. The condition of the mother and child is checked during the postpartum (after delivery) period; in some cases, the care of the newborn is referred to a pediatrician after a few days.

Gynecology is the study of *female* diseases and disorders of the female reproductive system. The practicing physician is a gynecologist. Frequently, the physician is both an obstetrician and a gynecologist and his medical practice is referred to as OB-GYN practice.

In many rural areas, the general practitioner handles all obstetrical and gynecological cases as well as caring for the newborn after delivery.

OPHTHALMOLOGY

Ophthalmology is the study of the diseases and disorders of the eye. The physician who practices ophthalmology is a licensed physician who has specialized in ophthalmology. He should not be confused with the optometrist or optician. An *ophthalmologist* diagnoses and treats diseases while an *optometrist* measures visual disorders and prescribes and makes eyeglasses to correct the visual problem. An optometrist is not a physician. An *optician* grinds lenses to the prescription ordered. He is not a physician either.

An ophthalmologist diagnoses eye conditions and treats them, frequently by surgical procedures. Some eye disorders that would be treated by an ophthalmologist are *presbyopia* (loss of elasticity of the lens) *myopia* (nearsightedness) *hyperopia* (farsightedness) *cataract* (opaque lens) *glaucoma* (increased intraocular pressure) and *keratitis* (inflammation of the cornea).

ORTHOPEDICS

Orthopedics is the study of the diseases and disorders of the bones of the body. The physician who practices orthopedic medicine is an orthopedist.

In addition to the treatment of fractures, the orthopedist is concerned with diagnosing and treating other types of bone disorders. Arthritis, degenerative joint diseases, bone tumors, osteomyelitis (inflammation of the bone) and low back pain are a few of the conditions seen and treated.

The practice of orthopedics may involve taking a great number of X rays for diagnoses and treatment. Also included is the application of casts and the insertion of pins in surgical procedures. Removal of pins in the office requires the preparation of a sterile setup. Preparation of a tray for the aspiration of fluid and joint injection, and measuring limbs of patients are other examples of procedures which the medical assistant will do.

PEDIATRICS

Pediatrics is the branch of medicine that deals with illnesses and health maintenance of children. The physician who practices pediatrics is a pediatrician.

The pediatrician practices preventive medicine as well as corrective medicine. Normal growth and development is a major concern in pediatrics. In addition to normal growth, the pediatrician administers the immunizations required during childhood. In a way, the pediatrician may be considered a generalist but restricts his practice to infants and children. He is a specialist in children's health and disorders.

PSYCHIATRY

Psychiatry is the study of disorders of the mind and emotions. The psychiatrist is a licensed physician who has specialized in psychiatry.

The *psychiatrist* diagnoses mental disorders and treats them in a variety of ways. Psychoanalysis is a longterm method of therapy in which the patient regresses through the past in order to find the cause of his illnesses. Chemotherapy (drug therapy) is frequently used in conjunction with other methods of psychotherapy. There are many schools of thought presently on the best method of therapy. Each psychiatrist will employ the method that he prefers.

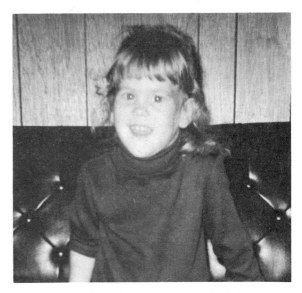

Normal growth and development of children is a major concern of pediatrics.

A *psychologist* is not a medical doctor but one who has recieved an academic degree from a school of higher learning and is involved mainly in measurement and testing of emotional stability.

SURGERY

There are many different types of surgery and many subdivisions in the specialty of surgery. If the physician specializes in *general surgery* he performs several kinds of surgery but mainly surgery of the internal organs.

There are many areas of specialty in surgery. Some of the areas are:

- Oral surgery
- Neurosurgery
- Plastic surgery
- Orthopedic surgery
- Gynecological surgery
- Cardiac surgery

Most of the specialty areas utilize surgical or operative techniques as a mode of treatment.

UROLOGY

Urology is the study of the diseases and disorders of the urinary tract. The practicing physician is a urologist. Urology, unlike gynecology, is concerned with the diagnoses and treatment of both male and female urinary tracts. It is also the specialty area that deals with male reproduction disorders or diseases.

Charts of Normal Values

Tests used to determine the presence or absence of various elements in the blood, stool and urine are outlined in charts on the following pages. Abbreviations used, as well as the complete name, identify the tests. The body fluid which is used, the required preparation, and the normal values provide reference information for the medical assistant.

Facts about X rays and temperature conversions, to simplify learning the metric equivalent of Fahrenheit readings, complete the appendix aids.

Blood Studies

BLOOD CHEMISTRIES

TEST	COMPLETE NAME OF TEST	BODY FLUID	PATIENT PREPARATION	NORMAL VALUES	COMMENTS
Cardiac Disease					
SGOT	Serum Glutamic Oxalacetic Transaminase	Serum	None	4 – 19 IU	
CPIC	Creatinine Phosphokinase	Serum	None	0 – 70 IU	
HBD	a-hydroxybutyrate dehydrogenase	Serum	None	Check values with particular lab used	
LDH	Lactic dehydrogenase	Serum	None	29 – 92 IU	
LDH Isoenzymes	Separates into fractions I, II, III, IV, V	Serum	None	Requires interpretation	
Liver Function					
SGPT	Serum Glutamic Pyruvic Transaminase	Serum	None	4 – 25 IU	
Bilirubin	Total Bilirubin	Serum	None	1.4 mg%	
	Direct Bilirubin	Serum	None	0.4 mg%	
BSP	Bromsulphalein	Serum	None	5% retention	
Alk. PO_4	Alkaline Phosphatase	Serum	None	13 – 41 IU	
T.P.	Total Protein	Serum	None	6.0 – 7.8 gm%	
Alb.	Albumin	Serum	None	3.2 – 4.5 gm%	
Glob.	Globulin	Serum	None	2.3 – 3.5 gm%	
A/G ratio	Albumin/Globulin ratio	Serum	None	1.0 – 2.0 : 1	
CCF	Cephalin Cholesterol Flocculation	Serum	None	24 hrs. = negative 48 hrs. = 2+	
Thymol Turb.	Thymol Turbidity	Serum	None	0 – 5 units	

BLOOD CHEMISTRIES (Con't)

TEST	COMPLETE NAME OF TEST	BODY FLUID	PATIENT PREPARATION	NORMAL VALUES	COMMENTS
SMA 12/60 includes the following	Sequential Multiple Autoanalyzer	Serum (2 ml)	Fasting		
Ca	Calcium			9 – 11 mg%	
FBS	Fasting Blood Sugar (Glucose)			60 – 110 mg%	
PO_4	Inorganic Phosphorous			3.0 – 4.5 mg%	
BUN	Blood Urea Nitrogen			8 – 22 mg%	
U.A.	Uric Acid			males 2.1 – 7.8 females 2.0 – 6.4	
Chol.	Cholesterol			150 – 300 mg%	
T.P.	Total Protein			6.8 gm%	
Alb.	Albumin			3.5 – 5.5 gm%	
Bili.	Total Bilirubin			1.4 mg%	
Alk. PO_4	Alkaline Phosphatase			30 – 85 mU/ml	
SGOT	Serum Glutamic Oxaloacetic Transaminase			10 – 50 mU/ml	
LDH	Lactic Dehydrogenase			90 – 200 mU/ml	
Kidney Function					
BUN	Blood Urea Nitrogen	Serum	None	10 – 18 mg%	
Creat.	Creatinine	Serum	None	0.2 – 1.0 mg%	
Creat. Cl.	Creatinine Clearance	Serum & Urine (timed)	Food & Water Height & Weight	72 – 141 ml/min.	
Uric Acid	Uric Acid	Serum	None	males 2.1 – 7.8 mg% females 2.0-6.4	
Na	Sodium	Serum or Plasma	None	133 – 148 mEq/L	
K	Potassium	Serum or Plasma	None	3.8 – 5.3 mEq/L	
Cl	Chloride	Serum or Plasma	None	100 – 106 mEq/L	
CO_2	Carbon Dioxide	Serum or Plasma	None	22 – 30 mEq/L	
Pancreas					
Amylase	Amylase	Serum, Urine, Peritoneal, Fluid	None	50 – 150 units (serum) 35 – 260 units (urine)	
Lipase	Lipase	Serum	None	0 – 1.5 units	
Lipids					
Total Lipids	Total lipids	Serum	Fasting	450 – 800 mg%	

BLOOD CHEMISTRIES (Con't)

TEST	COMPLETE NAME OF TEST	BODY FLUID	PATIENT PREPARATION	NORMAL VALUES	COMMENTS
Triglycerides	Triglycerides	Serum	Fasting	10 – 190 mg%	
Cholesterol	Cholesterol	Serum	Fasting	150 – 250 mg%	
Lipoprotein Electrophoresis	Separation into types: I, II, III, IV, & V. Alpha, Pre-Beta, Beta	Serum	Fasting	Requires interpretation by pathologist	
Prostate Acid PO_4	Acid Phosphatase	Serum	None	0.1 – 0.15 IU	
Miscellaneous					
Li	Lithium	Serum	None	0	
Fe	Iron	Serum	None	65 – 125 mcg	
TIBC	Total Iron Binding Capacity	Serum	None	300 – 340 mcg	

PEDIATRIC CHEMISTRY

TEST	COMPLETE NAME OF TEST	BODY FLUID	PATIENT PREPARATION	NORMAL VALUES	COMMENTS
Ca	Calcium	Serum		11-13 mg%	
P	Phosphorous	Serum		4-7 mg%	
Sweat Test	Sweat Test	Sweat Test	½ hour wait	70 mEq/L	
Trypsin	Trypsin Activity	Stool	nonsterile stool	2 – 4+	
Xylose Tolerance	Xylose Tolerance	Urine	N.P.O.; 5 hr pooled urine collection	6.5 – 1.2	
Salicylates (A.S.A.)	Acetyl-Salicylic Acid	Serum	None	None	
Bili.	Bilirubin	Serum	Heel stick under 3 wks.	5 mg%	
Protein Electrophoresis	Separated into: Albumin, Alpha$_1$, Alpha$_2$, Beta, and Gamma.	Serum	None	Alb 4.07 – 5.03 Alpha$_1$ 0.15 – 0.35 Alpha$_2$ 0.41 – 0.66 Beta 0.52 – 0.83 Gamma 0.45 – 0.66	(Normal values are based on full term infants at one year)
Immunoglobulins	Separates into A, D, M, G, E.	Serum	None		

COAGULATION

TEST	COMPLETE NAME OF TEST	REQUIRED BODY FLUID	PATIENT PREPARATION	NORMAL VALUES	COMMENTS
Fibrinogen level	Same	Plasma	None	200 – 400 mg%	
Protime	Prothrombin Time	Plasma	None	12 sec.	
PTT	Partial Thrombo-plastin Time	Plasma	None	35 sec.	
Bl. Time	Bleeding Time	Whole blood	Earlobe puncture	1 – 6 min.	
Cl. Time	Clotting Time	Whole blood	None	Each patient sets his own normal, usually 15 sec.	
Factor Assays	V, VII, VIII, IX, X XI, XII, XIII	Plasma			
Staph. Cl.	Staphylococcal Clumping	Plasma	None	6 mcg/ml	
Pro. Sulfate Dil.	Protamine Sulfate Dilution	Serum (treated)	None	negative	
Clot. Ret.	Clot Retraction	Whole blood		½ original mass in 1 hour.	

HEMATOLOGY

TEST	COMPLETE NAME OF TEST	REQUIRED BODY FLUID	PATIENT PREPARATION	NORMAL VALUES	COMMENTS
*CBC	Complete Blood Count	Whole blood	None		
*RBC	Red Blood Cell Count	Whole blood	None	male: 4.6-6.2 million female: 4.2-5.4 million	
*WBC	White Blood Cell Count	Whole blood	None	5 – 10,000	
*Plat	Platelet Count	Whole blood	None	150 – 450,000/ cu. mm	
*Hg	Hemoglobin	Whole blood	None	male: 14-18 gm female: 12-16 gm	
*Hct. or Crit.	Hematocrit	Whole blood	None	male: 40-54 vol% female: 37-47 vol%	
*Diff	Differential	Whole blood	None		
Eos	Eosinophils			1 – 4/100 WBC	
Baso	Basophils			0 – 1	
Segs PMN	Segmented Neutro-philic Granulocyte: Segmented Neutro-phil; or Polymor-phonuclear Neutro-phil			60 – 70	
Stabs	Single-lobed Neu-trophil Band			0 – 1	
Mono	Monocyte			2 – 6	
Lymphs	Lymphocytes			25 – 35	
*Retic Count	Reticulocyte Count	Whole blood	None	0.5 – 1.5	

*May be done on a finger, heel, or earlobe puncture. (Chart continued on page 238).

HEMATOLOGY (Con't)

TEST	COMPLETE NAME OF TEST	REQUIRED BODY FLUID	PATIENT PREPARATION	·NORMAL VALUES	COMMENTS
L.E. Cells	Lupus Erythematosus Cells	Whole blood	None	None	
Sickledex	Sickle Cell Screening Test	Whole blood	None	no sickling	
Sed Rate ESR	Sedimentation Rate Erythrocyte Sedimentation Rate	Whole blood	None	males: 15/hr females: 20/hr	
Cell Indices					
MCH	Mean Cell Hemoglobin	Whole blood	None	21-31 $\mu\mu$g (micromicrograms)	
MCV	Mean Cell Volume	Whole blood	None	82-92 cuμ (cubic microns)	
MCHC	Mean Cell Hemoglobin Concentration	Whole blood	None	32-36%	

SEROLOGY

TEST	COMPLETE NAME OF TEST	REQUIRED BODY FLUID	PATIENT PREPARATION	NORMAL VALUES	COMMENTS
STS	Standard Test for Syphilis	Serum	None	Nonreactive	Test which is standard in the particular laboratory will be performed
*RPR	Rapid Plasma Reagin	Serum	None	Nonreactive	
VDRL	Veneral Disease Research Laboratory	Serum	None	Nonreactive	
FTA	Fluorescent Treponemal Antibody	Serum	None	Nonreactive	
CRP	C-Reactive Protein	Serum	None	Negative	
ASO	Antistreptolysin-O Titer	Serum	None	1:166	
IM	Infectious mononucleosis	Serum	None	Negative	
RA **R_3**	Rheumatoid Arthritis R_3 Screen Test	Serum	None	Negative	

*May be done on a finger stick.

Skin and Stool

TEST	COMPLETE NAME OF TEST	REQUIRED BODY FLUID	PATIENT PREPARATION	NORMAL VALUES	COMMENTS
Skin Tests					
TBC	Tuberculosis	None	None		Intradermal injection
PPD-S	Purified Protein Derivative-Standard	None	None		Intradermal injection
PPD-B	-Battey				
Stool					
O & P	Ova & Parasites	Stool	None	Negative	
Scotch-Tape Test	Scotch-Tape Test	Anal tape	None	Negative	

Urine Studies

URINALYSIS (Routine, Microscopic)

TEST	COMPLETE NAME OF TEST	REQUIRED BODY FLUID	PATIENT PREPARATION	NORMAL VALUES	COMMENTS
Routine Ua consists of:	Routine Urinalysis	Urine	Random specimen	See details below under individual tests	
Sp. gr.	Specific Gravity			1:012 – 1.035	
Color	Color			Straw to light amber	
pH	Hydrogen + ion concentration			average = 6.0 range = 4.6 – 8.0	
Glucose	Glucose (dextrose)			None	
Ketones	Acetone, diacetic acid & Betahydroxy-butyric acid			None	
Hg.	Hemoglobinuria			None	
Bile	Bile			None	
Sq Epith Cells	Squamous Epithelial Cells			Occasional	
RBC	Red Blood Cells Hematuria			Occasional - none	
WBC	White Blood Cells			Occasional - none	
Crystals				Occasional	
Acid Urine	Calcium oxalate & carbonate, amorphous urates, uric acid				
Alkaline Urine	Amorphous phosphate, triple phosphates				
Flagellates	Trichomonas vaginalis			None	
Casts	Red Cell; White Cell; Coarsely granular; Finely granular; Waxy; Hyaline; Bacterial			no casts or rare hyaline cast with no cellular elements	
T.L.C.	Thin Layer Chromatography (for sugar identification)				

URINE CHEMISTRIES

TEST	COMPLETE NAME OF TEST	REQUIRED BODY FLUID	PATIENT PREPARATION	NORMAL VALUES	COMMENTS
Pregnancy Test	Two-hour Wampole Direct Agglutination Pregnancy Test (DAP) Pregnosticon	Urine	First morning specimen	None as such - depends on particular test	
Estriol	Placental Estriol		24 hour total volume	8 mg	
VMA	Vanillymandelic Acid		Special diet & 24 hour collection	1 – 8 mg/24 hrs.	
17 K.S.	17 Keto-steroids		24 hour collection	Female 6 – 12 mg	
17 Kg.S	17 Ketogenic Steroids			Male 8 – 15 mg.	
Amylase	Amylase		2 hour timed specimen or 24 hour collec.	35 – 260 units/hour	
5HIAA	5 hydroxyindole acetic acid		Random	Negative	
	Serotonin quantitative		24 hour collection.	16 mg	
Urine Electrolytes					
Na – K – Cl	Sodium		24 hour collection	130 – 260 mEq/24hr.	
	Potassium		24 hour collection	24 – 100 mEq	
	Chloride		24 hour collection	110 – 250 mEq	
Calcium	Sulkowitch		Random	1+	
PSP	Phenylsulfonphthalein		2 hr. test dye injection	15 min 25% 2 hrs. 70%	

Facts About X rays

BONY STRUCTURES

Any bone can be x-rayed from many different angles and planes: fetal bones can be x-rayed before birth to show viability and age of the fetus. No preparation is necessary except for Myelogram and Bronchogram.

Chest — Routinely done in PA (postero-anterior) and lateral positions. Other views are obliques, decubitus, expiratory, inspiratory, overexposure, AP supine and lordotic.

Bronchogram — special procedure which requires injection of contrast by a physician into bronchial tree — requires premedication of patient and post x-ray care.

Spine — Cervical — AP (antero-posterior), oblique, open-mouth
Thoracic (or dorsal) — AP, lateral, obliques
Lumbar — AP, lateral, oblique
Lumbo-sacral — AP, lateral, oblique
Sacrum and coccyx — AP, lateral

Myelogram — special x-ray procedure which requires injection of contrast in spine by physician. Requires premedication of patient; done on inpatient basis.

Skull — multiple views

Sinuses — paranasal sinuses taken in multiple views

Sinogram — injection of contrast by physician

GASTROINTESTINAL SYSTEM

Abdomen — flat plate, AP position; other views, decubitus, upright. No prep.

GI Series (colon and stomach) — requires 2 days with laxative enemas and fasting of patient.

Upper GI (esophagus and stomach) — drinking of contrast by patient during fluoroscopy to outline stomach; preparation of patient is by fasting.

Lower GI (colon or barium enema) — contrast given to patient by enema during fluoroscopy to outline the lower bowel; preparation of patient is by laxative and enemas.

GB (gallbladder series) — oral administration of contrast night before test; preparation of patient by eating fat-free diet night before and taking pills, fasting in morning before X ray is to be taken.

Barium Swallow (esophagram) — no patient preparation, contrast taken orally by patient during fluoroscopy.

Air-Contrast Enema — preparation of patient involves diet, laxative and enemas for several days in advance of test. Bowel is outlined by injection of air into lower bowel after barium.

Small Bowel series — preparation of patient is by fasting, oral administration of contrast to patient and X rays taken to follow contrast throughout the small bowel.

GENITO-URINARY SYSTEM

KUB (kidneys, ureters, bladder) — flat plate of abdomen — requires no prep.

IVP (intravenous pyelogram) — intravenous injection of contrast requires preparation of patient with laxative, enemas and fasting.

Voiding Cystogram — injection of contrast into bladder by catheter — no special preparation, often done in conjunction with IVP.

Retrograde Pyelogram — usually done in conjunction with cystoscopy, can be done as outpatient, requires patient preparation; injection of contrast into kidneys by urologist.

GYNECOLOGICAL SYSTEM

Abdomen — flat plate to determine number, position or age of fetus — no preparation.

Pelvimetry — AP and lateral position — to measure size of pelvis and fetus.

Salpingogram — injection of contrast into uterus and tubes for sterility workup by physician — preparation of patient requires laxatives, may be either inpatient or outpatient.

Mammography — X ray of breast — no preparation of patient.

SPECIAL STUDIES

Arteriograms
Venograms
Lymphangiograms } contrast is injected by physician under sterile conditions into an artery, vein or lymph vessel, usually for diagnostic purposes; requires premedication of patient and post X ray observation.

Laminogram — moving x-ray tube and film in opposite directions during exposure producing serial cuts of specific area, e.g. tumor of lung.

NUCLEAR MEDICINE

Scans — injection or ingestion of radioactive material which produces picture of almost any organ in body.

Uptake Studies — of thyroid gland.

Radioactive therapy — treating tumors and hyperthyroid with radiactive material.

Flow studies — radiology study of arteries and veins, lymph areas for diagnostic study.

RADIATION ONCOLOGY

Treatment of tumors using X rays or gamma rays.

Cobalt and radium or caesium sources.

Deep Therapy — Betatron or linear accelerator (very high energy)

TEMPERATURE CONVERSIONS FROM FAHRENHEIT TO CELSIUS (Metric)

The metric system is gradually replacing other systems of measurement. In order to convert Fahrenheit temperatures to Celsius temperatures, the following formula may be applied: (1) Subtract 32 from the Fahrenheit reading. (2) Multiply the result by 5/9.

The following chart may be used for quick reference.

°F	°C	°F	°C	°F	°C	°F	°C
70	21.1	117	47.2	160	71.1	197.6	92
71	21.7	118	47.8	161	71.7	198	92.2
72	22.2	119	48.3	161.6	72	199	92.8
73	22.8	120	48.9	162	72.2	199.4	93
74	23.3	121	49.4	163	72.8	200	93.3
75	23.9	122	50	163.4	73	201	93.9
76	24.4	123	50.6	164	73.3	201.2	94
77	25	124	51.1	165	73.9	202	94.4
78	25.6	125	51.7	165.2	74	203	95
79	26.1	126	52.2	166	74.4	204	95.6
80	26.7	127	52.8	167	75	204.8	96
81	27.2	128	53.3	168	75.6	205	96.1
82	27.8	129	53.9	168.8	76	206	96.7
83	28.3	129.2	54	169	76.1	206.6	97
84	28.9	130	54.4	170	76.7	207	97.2
85	29.4	131	55	170.6	77	208	97.8
86	30	132	55.6	171	77.2	208.4	98
87	30.6	132.8	56	172	77.8	209	98.3
88	31.1	133	56.1	172.4	78	210	98.9
89	31.7	134	56.7	173	78.3	211	99.4
90	32.2	135	57.2	174	78.9	212	100
91	32.8	136	57.8	174.2	79	213	100.6
92	33.3	136.4	58	175	79.4	214	101.1
93	33.9	137	58.3	176	80	215	101.7
94	34.4	138	58.9	177	80.6	215.6	102
95	35	139	59.4	177.8	81	216	102.2
96	35.6	140	60	178	81.1	217	102.8
96.8	36	141	60.6	179	81.7	218	103.3
97	36.1	141.8	61	179.6	82	219	103.9
98	36.7	142	61.1	180	82.2	219.2	104
98.6	37	143	61.7	181	82.8	220	104.4
99	37.2	144	62.2	181.4	83	221	105
100	37.8	145	62.8	182	83.3	225	107.2
100.4	38	145.4	63	183.2	84	230	110
101	38.3	146	63.3	184	84.4	235	112.8
102	38.9	147	63.9	185	85	239	115
102.2	39	147.2	64	186	85.6	240	115.6
103	39.4	148	64.4	186.8	86	245	118.3
104	40	149	65	187	86.1	248	120
105	40.6	150	65.6	188	86.7	250	121.1
105.8	41	150.8	66	188.6	87	255	123.9
106	41.1	151	66.1	189	87.2	257	125
107	41.7	152	66.7	190	87.8	260	126.7
107.6	42	152.6	67	190.4	88	265	129.4
108	42.2	153	67.2	191	88.3	266	130
109	42.8	154	67.8	192	88.9	270	132.2
110	43.3	154.4	68	192.2	89	275	135
111	43.9	155	68.3	193	89.4	280	137.8
112	44.4	156	68.9	194	90	284	140
113	45	156.2	69	195	90.6	285	140.6
114	45.6	157	69.4	195.8	91	290	143.3
115	46.1	158	70	196	91.1	295	146.1
116	46.7	159	70.6	197	91.7	300	148.9
116.6	47	159.8	71				

Acknowledgments

The author wishes to thank all who participated in the development of this text.

Reviewer

Mrs. Rose Hall, RN, CMA
Coordinator, Medical Assistant Program
Belleville Area College, Belleville, Illinois.

Contributions of Content and Illustration

The student medical office assistants at Athens Technical School.
Beverly Kissinger for various line drawings used throughout the text.
Each subject who consented to be included in the photographs.

American Optical Corp., figures 6-2, 31-4, 31-5.

American Hospital Supply Corp., figure 10-3.

Ames Company, figures 30-3, 4, 5, 6; 32-1, 2, 3, 4.

Athens Technical School, Figures 3-8, 3-10, 5-2, 11-1, 12-1, 13-1.

Baxter Laboratories, figure 12-3.

Becton-Dickinson, figures 20-2, 27-4.

Crisp County Hospital, Cordele, Ga., figures 3-9, 8-4, 12-2, 12-4, 17-5, 18-2, 3; 20-4, 28-3, 31-6, 34-1, 2; 35-1, 2, 3, 4, 5; 36-1, 2.

IVAC Corp., figure 3-5.

J.B. Lippincott Co., figures 16-1, 17-1, 4.

Professional Disposable Products, Inc., figure 12-5.

Ritter Equipment Co., figure 10-1.

Sherwood Medical Industries, Inc., figure 12-3.

Wyeth Co., figures 9-1, 2, 4; 10-2, 16-3.

Contributions by Delmar Staff

Publications Director — Alan N. Knofla
Source Editor — Angela R. Emmi
Copy Editor — Ruth Saur
Editorial Assistant — Peggy Vernieu
Director of Manufacturing and Production — Frederick Sharer
Illustrators — Tony Canabush, George Dowse, Mike Kokernak, Al DeBenedetto
Production Specialists — Debbie Monty, Patti Manuli, Betty Michelfelder, Sharon Lynch, Jean LeMorta, Alice Schielke, Lee St. Onge

Index

Sterile field, 69-72
Sterile objects, transfer of, 69-72
Sterilization, 45, 50-51
Sterilizer
  advantages, 61-62
  description, 61
  principles, 61
  use of, 62-63
Stethoscope, 16
Stimulants, 143-144
Stirrup position. *See* Dorsal recumbent position
Streptococci, 42
Subcutaneous injection, 157-158
Superficial heat, 106-107
Surface heat. *See* Superficial heat
Surgery, 233
Surgical asepsis, 69
Suture pack, 57
Syphilis tests, 200
Syrup of Ipecac, 146
Systemic infection, 44
Systole, 15
Systolic pressure, 16

T

Tachycardia, 14
Tapotement, 108-109
Telfa, 89
Temperature conversions, 243
Terpin hydrate, 146
Therapeutic, 124
Therapy, 124
Thermal rays, 107
Thermometers
  oral, 12
  rectal, 12
Tranquilizers, 145
Treatment
  cold application, 95
  dressings, 89-90
  heat applications, 93-95
  irrigations, 97-103
  minor surgery, assisting with, 77-80
  physical therapy, 106-109
Treatment room, preparing, 79

True proportions, 138

U

Urinalysis, routine, 176-180
Urine
  chemical examination, 177-178
  microscopic examination, 178-180
  physical examination of, 176-177
Urine specimens, 116-117
Urine studies, 239
Urine tests, 200
Urologist, 111
Urology, 233
Uterine bleeding, 220

V

Vaginal irrigation, 100-102
Vasodilators, 144
Venipuncture, 118
Vibration, 109
Vibrio, 42
Visual observation, 33
Vital signs
  blood pressure, 15-16
  pulse, 13-14
  respiration, 14-15
  temperature, 11-13
Vitamin K, 146
Vitamins, 146
Volumetric flasks, 169

W

Weight, 16-17
White blood cell count. *See* Leukocyte count
Wintrobe tube. *See* Hematocrit tube

X

X-ray examinations, 204-205
X rays, 202
  bony structures, 241
  gastrointestinal system, 241
  genito-urinary system, 242
  gynecological system, 242
  radiation oncology, 242
  special studies, 242
Xylocaine, 80